The Day Room

A Memoir of Madness and Mending

Kathleen Crowley

Kennedy Carlisle Publishing Co.
Madison, Wisconsin

Kennedy Carlisle Publishing Co.
630 South Whitney Way, Suite 120
Madison, WI 53711

Library of Congress Cataloging-in-Publication Data

Crowley, Kathleen, 1956-
The day room : a memoir of madness and mending / by Kathleen Crowley : with a foreword by Lee Jones, M.D. -- 1st ed.
p. cm.
Includes bibliographical references and index.
ISBN 0-9643348-0-1. -- ISBN 0-9643348-1-X (pbk.)
1. Crowley, Kathleen, 1956---Health. 2. Chronic pain--Patients--California--Biography. 3. Depressed persons--California--Biography. 4. Emergency medical personnel--California--Malpractice. I. Title.
RB127.C785 1995
616.85'27'0092--dc20
[B] 94-46756
CIP

ISBN: 0-9643348-0-1

0 9 8 7 6 5 4 3 2 1

Printed and bound in the United States of America.

This book is for my daughters Acasia and Amanda
in the hopes that they may better understand,
For my mother Peggy Crowley
because she always tried to,
And for Dr. Lee Jones and Dr. Bruce Oppenheim
because they always did.

KC

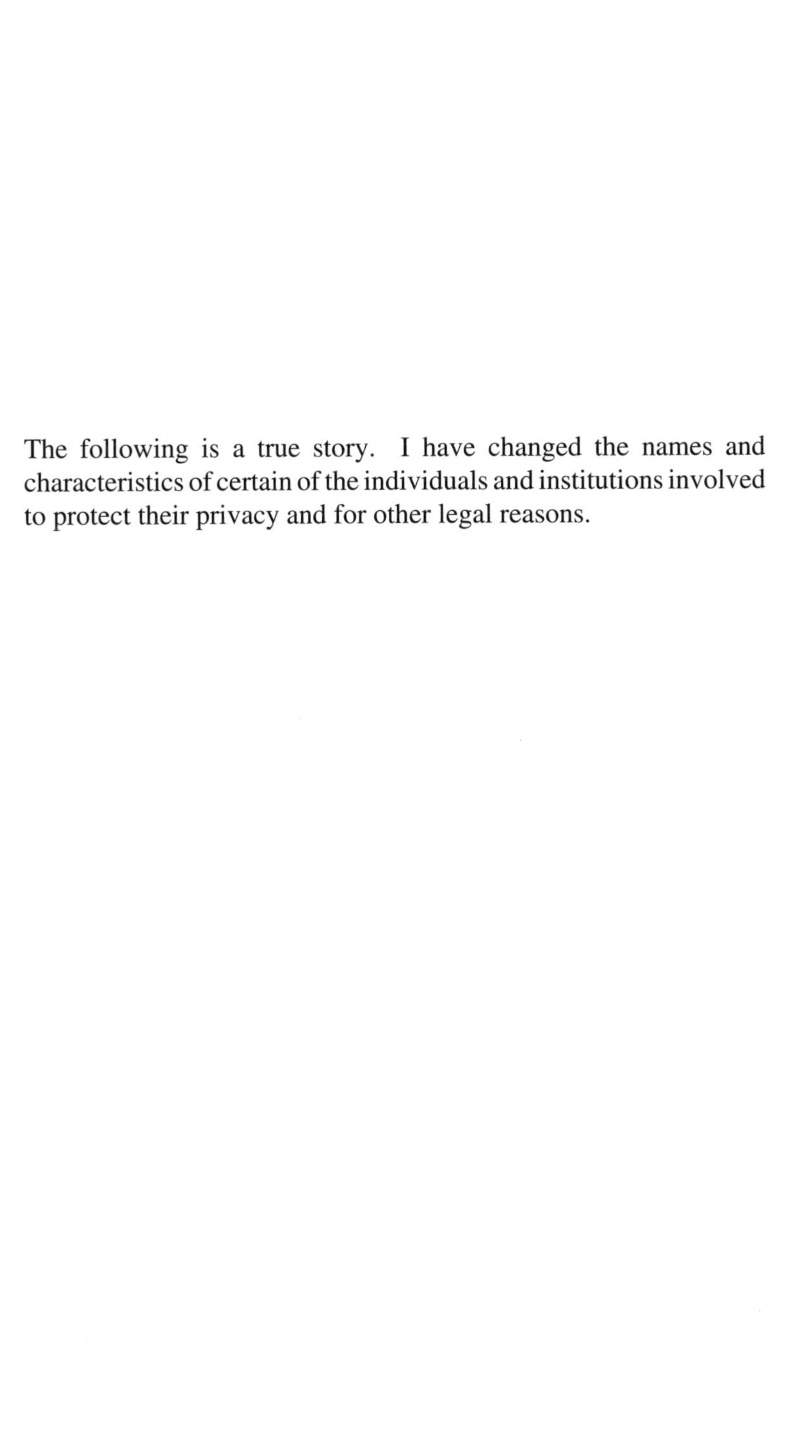

The following is a true story. I have changed the names and characteristics of certain of the individuals and institutions involved to protect their privacy and for other legal reasons.

Contents

Foreword

Human spirit is a very funny thing. It requires care, nurture, support and gentle guidance. It also needs freedom, to be allowed to let go of responsibilities, and even of reality at times. Too much of either direction or freedom and our spirit fails to thrive and withers. It's like a rosebush: fail to support it well and it won't grow tall and straight with many blossoms; support it too tightly and it's stunted. A fine balance is needed, and a good gardener knows that a variable mixture of sun, water, soil, wind, food, and protection is needed. So, the human spirit, like all living things, not only thrives on but needs many things for survival, and often these needs seem to contradict each other. This all sounds so complicated. But, as roses have been growing and thriving for centuries, perhaps none of this is as complicated as we fear.

Many times, and for as many different reasons as there are people, we get lost and our spirit suffers. Over the millennia our species has come up with many ways of trying to heal that suffering and find life's meaning. We've followed many religious leaders with their various ideologies in hopes that they will help us find our way. Nations, companies, and myriad organizations and institutions have formed in hopes that their identity will be our choice for external validity. Psychotherapies have developed in belief that we can change our internal validity. To varying degrees, these have been successful. But individual human beings suffer today unabated—physically and spiritually—no less than individual humans thousands of years ago. So can we realistically look to our institutions to solve human suffering?

I met Kathleen after she had seen dozens of doctors. She was in unimaginable physical pain likened to a war veteran with a bullet lodged in his spine. She was in a suicidal depression from a chemical imbalance resulting from her pain and worsened by the many doctors who diagnosed her problem as emotional. She'd built a wall around her, but early on she let me in. She might have committed suicide, or accepted the lifelong alternative of permanent disability, continued dependence on the medical profession and morphine that the institutions offered her. But at the critical point, she challenged her pain and her life and that made all the difference. *The Day Room* is her inspiring story.

As I review my years of treatment of patients around the country, with cancer, with AIDS, with transplants, with debilitating physical pain, I consider: what makes the difference? What aspects of human spirit open the doors to survival and mastery over suffering? I can think of three such aspects, all of which applied to Kathleen:

1. There is a tremendous instinct to close down; to build walls separating ourselves from the unjust world, to focus on the fact that life is not fair. The human spirit must be able to accept the unfairness of life, to tear down those walls; and as a result be able to clearly and analytically look at the world and the available choices.

2. Even in the midst of suffering, there must be trust and faith in another. It cannot be done alone, nor should it.

3. The human spirit must reach for health, as a plant reaches for light, not for others (i.e., not because of guilt) but for itself—based not only on a genuine feeling of self worth but also a genuine desire to live a meaningful life despite limitations.

When a child is lost in a forest, it is always a large organization that conducts the search; police, military, or rangers. On the news, we watch massive search and rescue operations complete with helicopters, planes, and infrared night glasses. But, when the child is rescued, it's not an army we see. One man or one woman carries the frightened child to safety. The massive effort comes down to a simple human interaction and a child finds the way home.

The Day Room is unique because from it we can see how we each can make a difference in our personal interactions—whether we're the doctor, the lawyer, the husband or wife, the friend or the patient.

Since what happened to Kathleen could have happened to your closest friend, your child, your lover or even you, you must read this book and learn its wonderful secrets. *The Day Room* is a remarkable personal account of a victory of the human spirit, and the insights and people that make the difference.

Lee Jones, M.D.
Los Angeles, California
September 1994

The Day Room

The Mystery of Pain

Pain has an element of blank
    It cannot recollect
When it began, or if there were
    A day when it was not.

It has no future but itself
Its infinite realms contain
Its past, enlightened to perceive
New periods of pain.

— *Emily Dickinson*

The Door

"There are things which must cause you to lose your reason, or you have none to lose."

— Gotthold Ephraim Lessing

I awoke at six in the morning, August 30th 1984. The alarm was blaring and I was reluctant to give up the escape I now so often sought in sleep. My suitcase in the corner of the room served as a chilling reminder of what the day was to hold. Mechanically I rose, showered, dressed and made coffee.

For two days I'd been cleaning, shopping, doing laundry, making lists. I wanted everything as organized as possible for my mother, who would be taking care of my daughters while I was away.

Acasia and Amanda were only three and five. It broke my heart to leave them. Slowly I wandered in to each of their bedrooms, and I gazed at them sleeping. They looked angelic and peaceful and terribly beautiful. I thought about the long talks that I'd had with them the previous evening. And I thought of the look of terror they both had on their faces at the time. Painfully, I turned away.

By now my husband Andrew was up, and as I was gathering all of my things together, he handed me a paperback book. "Here, I picked this up for you. I don't know anything about it but it looked interesting." Underneath a gruesome cover picture, I read in bold letters "IT ASSAILS ONE'S VERY GRIP ON REALITY."

I handed the book back to Andrew, staring at him, saying nothing.

"I don't know what's happened to you Kathy," he said sadly. "I just wish you were the way you used to be."

Ah well whoopee doo I thought, amused at the impossibility of his wish. I wish lady slippers grew freely by the side of the road and flamingos roamed the city. Of course I didn't say what I was thinking; I'd stopped doing that some time ago.

My mother arrived, breathless, nervous. Andrew carried my suitcase out. I kissed Amanda and Acasia, hugged them tight ... tighter.... kissed them again, acknowledged my mother in some way, and left. I will always remember the girls' two tiny figures standing there waving at me. Both of them strong and straight and brave. Amanda's arm around Acasia.

Andrew and I traveled in silence. Not a comfortable silence, but a now common one. When we arrived, suitcase and all, to the admitting area, the woman behind the counter said she had no admission instructions for me. She said in an impatient, sarcastic tone, "You know, you can't just walk in off the street and admit yourself to the hospital."

I wanted to say, "Look stupid, I have no great desire to stay here. This place that houses the very profession that I hate the most. The very profession that...." I wanted to say, "Fuck you. Your mother wears army boots." Instead I said "I spoke with Dr. Marks yesterday. He said he'd arranged for my admission." I gave her Dr. Marks' phone number and she excused herself to call him.

She soon returned. "Well, I left a message at his office. He's due in within the hour. Maybe you two would like to get some coffee in the meantime?"

As Andrew and I walked to the cafeteria, we felt angry. It seemed we were continually being faced with incompetence. Didn't they know we were at the end of our ability to cope? We agreed that if we returned to the admissions office and there was any further confusion, we'd forget this whole charade and return home. Ah home. What a comforting thought. I didn't feel comfortable for long though as I began to recall vividly the man's head on the fly's body in the old SciFi movie "The Fly." In a squeaky little sing song voice he cried, "Help me. Help me."

When we returned we were assured everything had been "taken care of" and that an escort would now be called for us. Our escort soon arrived, a nurse by the name of Ellen. Ellen was probably in her forties, with her hair in pig tails with bow ties, her blue jeans rolled up and two prominent circles of rouge on her cheeks. Terrific, I thought, chucko the clown for a nurse. Ellen watched me with what I felt was a mixture of compassion and curiosity, as the three of us proceeded down the long corridor. On the elevator Ellen began to chuckle and said with obvious amusement that she had just realized we must be wondering why she was dressed in that fashion. It was "Fifties Day" she said. The staff was having a party.

As we approached the ward door I hesitated. A sign on the door read, "CLOSE DOOR QUICKLY. ELOPEMENT RISK." Ellen unlocked the door. Andrew nudged me in. Once inside Ellen excused herself and we were left standing in a hall. Anxiously, awkwardly, unhappily. On each side of us was a room with patients. Straight ahead, completely enclosed, was the nursing station, which I later learned was commonly referred to by patients as "the cage."

A woman, close to fifty, with a mop of dark wavy hair and a lopsided grin approached me. She leered, seemingly interested in both Andrew and me, and introduced herself as Daisy. Daisy began to chatter, making little sense and after a couple of minutes reached out and began slowly and deliberately to finger my blouse.

"You're lovely," she said. "You look exactly like the one woman I *wish* was my mother."

I backed away. Minutes later, she reappeared as I was leaving the ladies room. With itsy bitsy spider movements, her fingers danced up my blouse. Cocking her head to one side, she smiled a wide, toothless grin.

I felt uneasy but at the same time numb.

Suddenly Daisy's fingers closed around my neck. "Don't be afraid," she whispered.

But I was. And as I darted out into the hall, she called, "They admitted the wrong one you know."

I found Andrew uncomfortably waiting for me. And as I relayed to him in my now customary monotone what happened, his voice grew loud. "She tried to choke you?" he shouted. "For God's sake Kathy, what are we doing?"

The only thing left, I thought, but said nothing.

We hesitantly seated ourselves in one of the two community

rooms, the "day" room. The room was furnished with large, ugly, orange vinyl couches and chairs, and a television was bolted into a wall cabinet with a stereo below. The day room was dark, dreary and depressing. How typical of the medical profession, I thought, to provide such a room.

Smoke and patients filled the room. One patient in particular sent a chill up my spine. He was stocky and muscular, probably in his twenties, and dressed entirely in black. He had short cropped blonde hair, and wore dark sunglasses. He moved constantly, rhythmic and catlike. He wore a Sony Walkman turned up full volume. He alternated between pacing back and forth in the hall and sitting in the day room staring. At me. It struck me that as slow and graceful as his movements were, he seemed full of rage, a volcano of fury that could erupt any time. He made no effort to conceal his staring at me. In fact, he removed his dark glasses to do so.

"Look at the way he is looking at me," I whispered to Andrew, "like he's going to murder me. "

"Not murder," Andrew said, "rape. Plain and simple. And *we* brought you here," he said, disgusted. "Where one woman's choking you and this guy is planning to rape you."

Smiling, Ellen popped her head into the day room and indicated that she would now show us to my room, and introduce me to my new roommate. Nancy was a thin, quiet woman; polite, reserved and not happy about sharing her room, I thought. Ellen mentioned in passing that Nancy was on "bed restriction," a statement that added to my already considerable anxiety. I wasn't familiar with "bed restriction" and could only imagine that I didn't want to be.

Andrew reluctantly said good-bye to me. He looked far older than his twenty-nine years and far sadder than I'd ever known him to be. And I felt extraordinarily guilty for involving him in all of this.

As he was just about ready to leave, he turned to me and said, with unusual feeling on his part, "This is horrible here Kathy and I know one thing for sure. *You* do not belong here."

I felt incapable of expressing any of the tenderness and concern I felt for him and instead I said, in a cold, desperate, angry tone, "That's the problem, isn't it Andrew? You tell me! Where the hell do I belong?"

Looking helpless, scared and defeated he turned to leave. I walked with him to the hall, at which point one of the nurses unlocked the door for him. And suddenly he was gone. And I was sorry. I wanted to call to him, to beg him not to leave me. I wanted so much for him to hold me, to tell me that everything was going to be all right. But I knew he couldn't help me any more. And I wasn't at all sure that anyone could. That was why I had, one hour earlier, signed myself into a locked psychiatric ward.

"Patient is a well groomed, well dressed white female who showed an appropriate amount of body movement. She was oriented times four. Memory was three out of three objects. Presidents: Reagan through Kennedy without difficulty. Five digits forward, three back. Thought: patient denies hallucinations, tangentiality or pressured speech. There was positive suicidal ideation. Proverbs were abstract. Similarities were abstract. Judgment good. Insight good."

— *Dr. Lee Jones, mental status examination on admission*

"Emotionally there is a certain coldness and distance to her."

— *Dr. Wilhelm Payne, defense psychiatrist*

I felt terribly afraid and I knew one thing for certain. I did *not* want to appear that way. I wanted to look confident and in control for the same reason I knew you should never let an animal sense your fear. You fall easy prey.

Hurriedly I returned to my room, in need of the privacy and safety I felt therein. I sat on the edge of the bed stiffly, and I waited—for what I had no idea.

After some time Ellen entered the room with two men. Mark Morris was a med student and Dr. Lee Jones was assigned to be my doctor for the length of my admission.

We all walked to Dr. Jones' office, which was outside of the ward, just down the hall. The office was small with no windows and no charm but just being away from the ward, even that small distance, felt better to me.

Next I was interviewed and asked questions that had my mind quickly wandering. "If you found a stamped, unmailed letter on the street, what would you do with it?" "If while a patron in a crowded movie theater, you suspected a bomb, what would you do?"

Sit and wait, I thought. "I would calmly let the manager of the theater know," I said.

It struck me that, as usual, they were making a stressful situation more so. What the hell did they hope to accomplish by badgering me? Why complicate things? Why not just talk to me? And not in riddles!

"What does, 'A rolling stone gathers no moss' mean?" Ditto: "People in glass houses shouldn't throw stones." "Count backwards from one hundred, by seven's." "Name the last five U.S. Presidents."

"Reagan, Carter, Nixon, Johnson, Kennedy... No, no, Ford goes in between Carter and Nixon," I said nervously. Great, I thought. I was satisfied that I even knew who the hell I was and they wanted to quiz me as if I was a contestant for a game show.

Dr. Jones, sensing my tension, laughed. "That's O.K. Everybody always forgets Ford."

I remember thinking that I'd begun doubting my sanity because everyone else seemed to be. Dr. Jones seemed to find nothing I said or did particularly unusual, or more important, a sign of "mental illness."

After a while I began to see some humor in the whole ridiculous situation. How amusing. This is good fun, I thought; I wonder when I get to do basket weaving. I love baskets.

"Tell me what brought you here," they wanted to know. My husband and his truck I thought.

"Well," I began to explain, "I was seen here at the U.C.L.A. Pain Clinic two weeks ago. They seem confident that they can alleviate my pain to some extent, but they have no idea how much, and they think that I'm too depressed to work with at this time. They want to see some improvement in my depression before they begin any treatments."

I began to feel full of the anger, the absolute fury that was now with me so much of the time. I said that I thought that this plan of action was absurd, that I was depressed because I hurt. If I didn't hurt I wouldn't be depressed and as long as I did I would. Why deal with the symptom? Why not the cause?

To my complete surprise Dr. Jones didn't interrupt me, nor did he give me the impression that he had far better things to do and that I was wasting his time. Instead he listened to me. Quietly and calmly he simply sat and listened to me. Am I in the Twilight Zone? I began to wonder. Doesn't this person realize that as a member of the medical establishment he is supposed to say specific things to me at this time? Things meant to reduce my level of self confidence while at the same time causing me to regard him as some type of God so that I would be a cooperative patient? A cooperative patient being one that is quiet, non-assertive, non-questioning, and perhaps most important one that readily pays his bill when it comes time.

My thoughts were interrupted by the unwelcome announcement that I was now to have a complete physical exam. I hated these! I felt like a pin cushion, a guinea pig, a piece of meat. My anxiety began to build. Once I was undressed and in a hospital gown I only felt worse. As a patient at a teaching hospital I knew that they would be learning on me. I felt frustrated and alone. And I felt violated.

As Mark was examining me, Ellen stood smiling warmly at me. I looked over at Dr. Jones standing in the corner of the small room. He was quietly observing Mark perform the exam. I thought about how, when Dr. Jones had first entered my hospital room and extended his hand to me, I'd felt an immediate and enormous sense of relief. He struck me as being both professional and appropriate, but more important and most surprising to me at that time, I just felt terribly glad that he was there.

Injection

Two and a half years earlier, April 29th 1982: Ten days after Acasia's first birthday. Andrew, the girls, my brother and I piled into my brother's old, beat up VW bug and went off to a local, inexpensive Mexican restaurant for dinner. Hours later, at home, I became dizzy, nauseous, hot, cold. I began vomiting, had diarrhea, and grew increasingly weak. Food poisoning? I wondered. I was the only one to eat a chicken burrito at dinner. I was concerned, since I was breast feeding Acasia at the time, that perhaps she too would become ill. If I was this sick I worried, what about her?

Andrew called a local hospital consistently recommended by the girls' pediatrician as "the one to call" in case of emergency. He was told that it sounded like flu symptoms but that without examining me it was anyone's guess. And so one by one Andrew carried us out to the car; two sleepy little girls and me, too weak and sick to walk.

Having been alerted by Andrew, a hospital attendant met us in the parking lot and wheeled me into the emergency room. From across the room someone called out disbelievingly, "You woke your kids up in the middle of the night for this? You just have the flu!"

A nurse appeared. She was small and attractive, probably about thirty-five years old with blue eyes, short blonde hair pulled back in a ponytail with a big pink bow, and a charm bracelet with dozens of charms. She laughed and shook her head, "I can't believe you'd get your kids up in the middle of the night for this!"

Andrew led the girls out to a bench in the corridor and the nurse wheeled me into an examining room. "You have the flu," she said, "You'll need an injection. The doctor will be here in a few minutes, and he'll tell you the same thing."

"If it's only the flu," I said, "I don't want an injection."

She sighed.

"I'm breast feeding," I said. "I don't want unnecessary medication."

"Well, you can discuss that with the doctor." As the door closed I heard footsteps approaching and the nurse say, "She's got the flu."

"O.K., get 50 mils of Phenergan."

"She's breast feeding."

"Make it 25." The door opened and there smiling stood the doctor. Energetically, cheerfully, he said, "Well, feel like you've got the flu?"

"I don't know what I feel like," I said. "I've never felt like this. I'm afraid I might have food poisoning, or appendicitis."

"Oh," he said smiling, "no chance of that. If you had either one you wouldn't be able to sit here like this."

"I've never felt like this with the flu," I said weakly.

"Well, it's a bad strain going around. We'll give you an injection and you'll be fine."

"Aren't you even going to examine me?" I asked.

His hand on the doorknob, he turned. "You want me to examine you? Fine, I'll examine you." He placed two fingers on my abdomen lightly. "Well, it does seem a bit..." I couldn't make out what he said. "But no," he said decisively, "no, you have the flu. We'll get you that injection and you'll be fine."

"I don't want an injection if it's only the flu," I said. "I'm breast feeding."

"Don't worry about that," he assured me.

"I am worried about that."

"Look, this is a really bad strain going around," he said. "You would probably be sick for three weeks without this injection."

"Well then," I said hesitating, "I'd like you to call Dr. Kohn, my pediatrician."

"No," he said. "There's no need for that."

I wasn't sure what to do. I wanted to feel better, but not at Acasia's expense. "But Dr. Kohn has always told me to check with him before taking any medication for as long as I'm breast feeding. He won't mind you calling him."

"No, no." And then as though conveying the strictest of confidence, he said softly, leaning towards me, "Trust me. I'm a pediatrician on the side."

"My husband was just promoted. He can't miss work. If you give me the injection, how soon will I be functional?"

"What is it that you do?" he asked thoughtfully.

"I have two small daughters, one and three. I have to be able to take care of them."

"You'll be fine in the morning," he said. "No problem." Opening the door, he nodded towards the nurse there waiting. "I'll let her do this, she's a pro." And then smiling, "She loves these."

Pain seared through me and I broke into a cold sweat. "Something is wrong," I whispered, terrified.

"Oh no," the nurse said assuredly. "These injections are painful. But they work. Now get dressed."

Dressed? I could barely move. I thought of how the needle hurt going in, and how long it seemed to have taken and how she'd wiggled it around and sighed, seeming frustrated.

Andrew had already gone to pull the car around. I again stammered to the nurse, "Something is wrong."

"Look I know the injection was painful but it will help. Now, you might want to have someone with you tomorrow," she said softening for the first time. "You'll probably be pretty out of it. Your daughters are beautiful," she said, as she sat waiting with me for Andrew to return. "I have four boys. I always wanted a daughter."

"Well you may have one yet," I said distracted.

"No, I won't. I'm separated from my second husband, I've had a hysterectomy, and anyway, I can't afford any more kids. I work three jobs as it is. If the hospital knew, they'd probably fire me. I haven't slept in seventy two hours, and I leave at the end of this shift, straight from the hospital, for a ski trip. I'm going with a man I've been seeing for a while now. Where I'll find the energy to ski, I don't know. I try to find the time to date but it's hard," she said looking worn and depressed. "It's so hard...."

One week later, May 7th, 1982 : At the girl's pediatrician for a routine visit, I described to Dr. Kohn how incredibly painful the injection had been, and the continued burning, hypersensitivity and pain since. I told him of the nurse's abruptness and lack of concern, and of the doctor's hurried "exam."

He asked who'd administered the injection, physician or nurse. And then he asked me to show him precisely the location of the injection. "Well, it seems a bit high....but I don't know," he said looking concerned. "It sounds like muscle damage to me. I think you should definitely see someone."

I'd only wondered when I could expect all of this to go away of its own accord. It hadn't entered my mind that it might not.

Dr. Kohn excused himself. I overheard bits and pieces of a phone call he placed; his voice raised, he sounded angry. He returned apologizing profusely on behalf of the hospital he had recommended. He said he'd just called Dr. Roosevelt Boxer, chief of staff of the emergency room. That Dr. Boxer would be getting in touch with me, and that they would certainly take care of me seeing someone.

A few days went by, the pain continued. No one from the hospital called me, so I called Dr. Boxer. "O.K.," he said, "let me get hold of your file, talk to the staff on duty that evening and get back to you."

About an hour and a half later he called. He said that he'd spoken to both the treating physician and nurse and that although neither of them had any recollection of me personally, they were both taken aback to find that anyone was less than one hundred per cent happy with their care. "And in that vein Mrs. Waddick, we'd like you to disregard the physician's fee, and only pay for your medication and the standard hospital emergency room portion of the bill, as we feel your care was standard and appropriate, but that you were not extended the *courtesy* you should have been. Regarding the injection having been ordered before the doctor examined you, that is standard hospital procedure. The emergency room is a busy place, as I'm sure you witnessed. Our nurses are well trained and to save time and lives, it is common for them to follow this procedure, the ordering of medication beforehand."

"Except," I said, "I was the only patient present at the time. If it's standard hospital procedure, that's fine. But the doctor should certainly follow up with an exam and confirm the diagnosis, don't you agree?"

After a long pause, he sighed and said, "Their actions were entirely appropriate Mrs. Waddick. What was inappropriate was that you overheard them. As a layperson I know that's difficult for you to understand, but the hospital is currently under construction, and we're temporarily lacking the necessary soundproofing. Now about this pain Mrs. Waddick, where are you experiencing this pain?"

"Where I had the injection."

Another long pause. "Which side of your body Mrs. Waddick?"

"The left."

"The left? Well there you have it Mrs. Waddick, whatever problems you are experiencing are entirely, without a doubt, unrelated to the Phenergan injection. Now you're more than welcome to seek any outside opinion you so desire, and I'd be interested in hearing the result. But in fact, you received the injection on the right."

"On the right? No, no, I didn't. It was the left."

"I have your file here Mrs. Waddick and our records clearly indicate the injection was given on the right."

"That is *not* so Dr. Boxer," I said stunned.

"In fact it is Mrs. Waddick. And I have the records to prove it. Good-bye Mrs. Waddick....and good luck."

On the right? He'd said *on the right*? And "the records to prove it?" What the hell was going on?

I wished that I had a family doctor to see. Someone who knew me. I'd been covered by a group medical plan while living with my parents before I married, a health maintenance organization where you rarely saw the same doctor twice. And other than for childbirth I'd had little cause to seek medical attention since.

The next day a neighbor told me of a "wonderful" general practitioner in the neighborhood. I called his office that afternoon and scheduled an appointment for the following day.

I liked Dr. Alexander. He appeared to be in his mid-fifties; handsome, friendly, self assured. He asked questions, made notes, and examined me. "You have a lot going on," he said gently. "You're all tied up in knots." He'd ordinarily prescribe a muscle relaxant, he said, but since I was breast feeding he'd have to use a more "conservative" approach.

"What is it that's wrong?"

"Well I can't be sure," he said. "But we'll fix you up. I have a variety of therapies we can try. You'll be fine," he said smiling gently as he gave my arm a squeeze. "I promise."

Thoughts of Marcus Welby came to mind, and I felt myself calming down.

Two-and-a-half months later, July 1982: I found myself no longer calmed by Dr. Alexander; his gentle manner, his promises, or his likeness to Marcus Welby. I now found his air of confidence appalling, maddening in fact.

He'd always denied any possible correlation between the injection and the pain while at the same time assuring me he knew both "just what was going on" and how to alleviate the pain entirely. So while I knew the injection had caused all of this, I didn't care whether or not he recognized this, as long as the end result would be the elimination of pain.

But I no longer felt confident that he knew "just what was going on." The area where I'd had the injection was horribly sensitive to the touch, and yet numb. It made no sense to me that it could be both, but it was. And in addition I was experiencing a multitude of different kinds of intense pain. Stabbing, shooting, burning, cramping, throbbing. I'd never experienced anything at all like this before and I felt at a complete loss.

So I asked Dr. Alexander again. Why wasn't I feeling better? In fact, why, after two months, did I only feel worse?

He led me to his office, took my hand in his and took a deep breath. "It is common," he said, "for young women with small children to feel exhausted, neglected, depressed. To feel that it's all too much for them. You tell your husband Mrs. Waddick," his voice stern, full of authority, "that I said you need some time away."

"Time away? Dr. Alexander, you said you could alleviate the pain. That's what I need."

He sighed and said softly, hesitantly, "I think it's emotional."

"You think it's what?" I gasped.

"The problem Mrs. Waddick, is that I just can't find anything wrong with you."

I just can't find anything wrong with you, I repeated to myself, trying to make some sense of the words. "Tell me Dr. Alexander, how it is then that you've been 'treating' me, administering physical therapy and assuring me that you would alleviate the pain all this time, and you think it's *emotional*?"

"Mrs. Waddick please, you're getting upset. Listen to me," he said. "You need a vacation." And then as if speaking to a child, "Now why don't you go home, tell your husband you need some time away, and try to relax."

"Relax? Dr. Alexander I'm in more pain than I ever thought

humanly possible. I feel like I'm losing my mind. I can't stand it anymore. I won't be able to relax 'away' any better than I can now."

Cutting me off, he said, "Mrs. Waddick, you're visibly upset. Now please go home, try to calm down, and think about what I've said."

I arrived home sobbing.

Andrew held me tight, and stroked my hair. "Kathy listen — Dr. Alexander obviously believed he could do something in the beginning, and when he couldn't help you, he needed an out. You need a specialist," he said. "We just need to locate the right doctor."

Doctors

A 92 year old man visited his doctor complaining of pain in his right knee.

"With your age," said the doctor, "what do you expect?"

"I don't know," said the man. "My left knee is also 92. But it feels great. So you tell me, what should *I expect?"*

— Michael McGarvey, M.D.

The next morning I called Dr. Kohn for a referral. His office suggested Dr. Leonard Shein, an orthopedic surgeon in the office building next to Columbus Memorial Hospital. Dr. Shein examined me as Dr. Alexander had, and then asked me to do a number of simple exercises—touch my toes; close my eyes and touch my nose; walk across the room normally, on my toes, then on my heels. Then he told me to dress and said he'd return in a few minutes to discuss his diagnosis.

"Early disc disease." My discs were thinning, he said, and would only deteriorate with time. He said there was no cure, no real treatment, and that my only line of action could be to attempt to "slow the process." He gave me a sheet of daily exercises to strengthen my abdominal muscles, and said that I'd need to rearrange my life accordingly. That I should refrain from all lifting, of children, groceries, etc. No bending. No heavy housework. No gardening. And definitely no leaning over to get children in and out of car safety seats.

"Your pain is completely unrelated to the injection, Mrs. Waddick. Columbus Memorial is a highly respected hospital. They know what they're doing over there," he said pointing to the hospital next door. "I can tell you that."

"But Dr. Shein," I said, "this all began at the time of the injection. I've never had any previous pain."

"I'm sure that you'd been experiencing pain for quite some time before the injection Mrs. Waddick. You just weren't aware of it."

"Not aware of it?" I repeated incredulously. "Dr. Shein, this pain is horrible. There's not a chance in hell I could have been unaware of it."

"Well, it's a slow process, Mrs. Waddick. The pain only recently built to this level and it just so happens that you had the injection right around the same time. Your pain and the injection are entirely unrelated."

I returned to my car where my friend Carla was waiting with the girls, who were asleep in their car seats, and I burst into tears. Looking at the girls, I began thinking about the changes in lifestyle Dr. Shein had prescribed for me. How was I to continue to care for the girls and Andrew and the house with such limitations? My days were currently full of prescribed "no-no's." I was forever popping the girls in and out of their car seats. And lifting and bending and cleaning and gardening. Andrew and I weren't in any position to have someone else do these things. He worked ridiculously long hours as it was so that we could get ahead. What's worse: Dr. Shein had predicted a lifetime of pain for me. The girls were only one and three. I was only twenty five. What was I to do?

More important, I knew that the pain was a direct result of the injection. I didn't buy the thinning disc theory. I was aggravated that anyone else did. And I was angry that I couldn't get anyone to listen to me.

Now what? I had Dr. Alexander telling me it was all in my head, and Dr. Shein (after reviewing the same x-ray's Dr. Alexander had) telling me I had early disc disease. And now nearly three months since the injection, three months of chronic pain, I wasn't sleeping and I wasn't eating. I was, in fact, a nervous wreck.

I rarely left the house any more. I couldn't bear to have clothes, or anything else, touch the area where I'd had the injection. The pain I was experiencing was "weird" pain. Indescribable pain. Yet I was always asked to describe it. "It burns. It sizzles…I have shooting pains and vise-like cramps. It throbs and tingles."

"Well, now that's a most unusual description, wouldn't you say, Mrs. Waddick?"

The little sleep I was now getting was continually interrupted by both pain and terrifying nightmares that had come to accompany it.

Relaying all this to my mother late one night, I burst into tears. My mother, full of anger and concern, suggested I see an attorney. An attorney? "Oh for goodness sake honey!" she said. "Something is WRONG here. This all began with the injection, and I think you should see an attorney about filing a lawsuit."

"I can't sue the hospital!" I said, surprised my own mother would suggest such a thing.

"Up until now I'd have agreed with you," she said emotionally, "But haven't you wondered why you can't find a doctor to treat you?"

Neil Newson, an attorney my mother had become friendly with over the past several years, called me the next afternoon. He was straightforward, all business. Neil suggested he send me to see someone and that with the doctor's report in hand, we'd talk. I agreed, relieved by the relative simplicity of this.

Days later, in the waiting room of the clinic Neil had referred me to, I didn't know what to think. This clinic was crowded, noisy, rundown. I felt angry. I couldn't believe that Neil would send me to such a place and I began to wonder if perhaps these doctors were paid to testify, rather than treat. Maybe, in fact, it was a scam. Maybe, I thought, only losers, only doctors that couldn't cut it in the real world would choose to work at such a place.

I was soon called in to see Dr. Jacoby, the clinic's orthopedic surgeon. He found absolutely nothing wrong, he said. He seemed apologetic but anxious to get on to the next patient. The waiting room was packed.

I felt close to tears. Gritting my teeth, and doing everything I could to remain rational, I said, "Dr. Jacoby, wait! I need help. I don't know what to do. Ever since I had the injection months ago I've been in pain. I know I 'look' fine, I 'walk' fine, I 'seem' fine. I hear that every day. But I'm not! I'm on edge. I can't sleep. I'm short tempered. I can't keep up with, let alone enjoy, my kids. And my husband and I no longer have any life together at all. This would all be hard enough if I knew what was wrong…but I can't deal with being told nothing. I wake up at night dripping with sweat and tears, from terrifying nightmares, screaming because I'm on fire, until I'm conscious enough to realize the fire is the burning where I had the injection. And I have cramping and stabbing and shooting pains so intense that at times I think I'd honestly rather be paralyzed. And where I had the injection, the skin is so sensitive to the touch that if a sheet lightly touches it at night it feels as if sand is being rubbed into a severe sunburn, never mind the irritation of wearing clothes. And so I stay home, wearing big loose dresses and nothing else, thinking I'm going to lose my mind and what's worse is that one by one you all sit across from me and calmly tell me nothing is wrong! Well, I'm telling you something is. And that the injection did it. And that I'm trying to find out what, and fix it, before I have a fucking nervous breakdown."

Dr. Jacoby looked away, and then spoke slowly, seeming to weigh each word carefully. "Mrs. Waddick, I want to help. I believe you're in pain—I just don't know why! And I don't know how to help." After a considerable pause he said gently, "I'll arrange for you to see one of our neurologists. I really don't think he'll be able to do much for you. But I just can't think of anything else to try."

Dr. Christian, the clinic's neurologist, was small-framed, pasty-complected, soft-spoken. His examination differed from others I'd had. It was more intense, involving new instruments, new questions and far more time.

"Sensory nerve damage, with the possibility of other complications as well," he said leaning back in his chair at the completion of his exam.

A wave of relief spread over me. I now had a name for all this pain. I felt validated. After a few minutes I asked smiling, "O.K. Dr. Christian, so what do I do now?"

No response.

"About this pain," I added.

"I don't think there's much you can do," he said.

"What do you mean? Now that I know what's wrong, I want to fix it!"

"I imagine you do," he said slowly, "but unfortunately only time will tell. Phenergan is a highly irritating medication and deep intramuscular penetration is mandatory to prevent injury to the skin and neighboring structures. Otherwise, as in your case, a variety of problems can arise. And it seems from the description of the pain you're experiencing that scar tissue may be an issue. I'm hoping it isn't, but only time will tell. Now nerves can and will," he continued, "attempt to regenerate themselves for up to eighteen months after injury. I want you to begin immediately taking Thiamine, vitamin B-1. It sometimes helps. I've written here for you the prescribed dosage. At some point down the line it might be appropriate for you to see a neurosurgeon or anesthesiologist, regarding the possibility of a nerve block."

"A nerve block?" I repeated slowly.

"Yes, an injection of alcohol or another pain suppressant into the nerve."

"An injection —" I chilled at the thought.

"Yes, but we don't need to discuss this today. Now pick some B-1 up and let's hope," he said opening the door.

"It is well-established that the mere fact of knowing what hurts you has an inherent cumulative value."

— *Hans Selye, M.D.*, The Stress of Life

He may think only time will tell, but I don't, I thought driving home. Now that I know the diagnosis, I can deal with it!

It felt so good not to be told that nothing was wrong, or that it was "early disc disease," or that yes, there's a problem, an emotional one. Having a name for the problem helped. I picked up the B-1 that night, feeling happy and confident that I was finally on the upswing.

That night at dinner Amanda picked up on my good mood. "Did the doctor fix you today, Mommy?" she asked happily. She stared at me intently, waiting.

"No, honey, he didn't fix me but ..."

"But mommy, you've been sick for so long."

"How long has it been?" Andrew asked quietly.

"I don't know. Four months?" I answered feeling suddenly defensive, guilty.

Amanda had tears streaming down her face. "I thought he'd make you back the way you were. I thought he'd fix you."

"Well, he didn't fix me, Amanda, but he did figure out what was wrong with me."

"And that's why you're so happy?" she asked, looking confused.

"Well, you can't fix something until you know what's wrong, honey."

"Are those pills going to fix you, Mommy?"

"They're vitamins, honey. They should help."

"Well then I want to take them too," she said emphatically, "so that never happens to me."

"Well, what about this nerve block thing?" Andrew said. "That might be good."

"A needle *good*? Do you remember that an injection created this whole mess, Andrew? And you think it might be a good idea?"

"Kathy, I know you're afraid. But it's not only *your* fear you need to consider. Look what this is doing to us—to all of us."

Soon the area where I'd had the injection began to itch profusely. This pleased me. The pain continued but I was hopeful now, which made a marked difference in my tolerance of it.

About a month later I returned to Dr. Christian's office smiling. "I am so itchy where I had the injection," I said excitedly, "isn't that a sign of healing?"

"Generally speaking yes," he said. He examined me, finding the numb area having decreased in size. "But nerves are so unpredictable," he continued. "Time is the only real indicator of how well you'll heal."

In the months to come my optimism began to dim. It was hard for me to keep my spirits up. The pain hadn't improved.

In desperation I called Neil.

He knew of "one of the best neurosurgeons in town," he said—the catch being "he won't testify." I made an appointment.

"You understand," Dr. Daniels said as he introduced himself, "that I am not going to testify in your lawsuit."

I nodded. "Neil told me this. The way I see it, if you can alleviate the pain, there won't be need for a lawsuit."

Dr. Daniels was likable, his examination seemed thorough, and Andrew and I waited breathlessly for his opinion.

"I have no doubt," he said, "that the pain you are experiencing is a result of the Phenergan injection."

"What can you do about it?" I asked.

"Mrs. Waddick, only time will tell." He gave me the same speech Dr. Christian had about the possibility of nerves regenerating themselves.

"What can you do about it now?" I asked shakily.

"Mrs. Waddick, the only known treatment is surgery, which in this case carries great risk. My guess is that scar tissue has formed and is now both entangled in and strangling other nerves. We would have to cut out the scar tissue, possibly doing further damage. You would, at best, have a large numb area."

"A large numb area? Sounds good to me. Right now, I have a large incredibly painful area."

"It's too risky," he said shaking his head.

"Dr. Daniels, I want surgery. It's my risk, and I'm willing to take it."

"Mr. Waddick," he said slowly, turning to Andrew, "listen to me. No experienced neurosurgeon is going to perform surgery at this time. If it were my own wife, I would not allow this surgery."

"Why? How much worse could I be?" I interrupted.

Dr. Daniels smiled at me. "Mrs. Waddick, you walked in here today. Imagine *not* being able to. If when it's been a considerably longer period of time, say 18 months, you feel the same you might consider it. At this time surgery would be unreasonably risky and any surgeon that would attempt it —"

"If I wait, in 18 months will *you* perform the surgery?"

Dr. Daniels bristled. "Mrs. Waddick, be reasonable. By performing this surgery, I would become involved in your lawsuit. You knew when you came in that I am not willing to testify. I'd have no choice if I was subpoenaed, which would certainly happen if I was your surgeon. I simply cannot risk my practice for someone's lawsuit. Have you any idea of the reaction from my colleagues and the American Medical Association? No doctor in his right mind will testify against another doctor or a hospital."

Is that what it came down to? I wondered. Was it too risky for me—or for him?

I began to cry.

"Doctors are men who prescribe medicines of which they know little, to cure diseases of which they know less, in human beings of whom they know nothing."

— *Voltaire*

I saw more doctors, doctors referred to me by doctors, and doctors referred to me by Neil. All agreed something was wrong, none agreed as to what. And no one knew how to help. Most were more than willing to write me prescriptions for pain pills however. I always asked about these pills that they seemed a little too anxious to prescribe.

"Mrs. Waddick," they would say, "anyone in the amount of pain you're expressing would do anything to alleviate it. Why all the questions?"

I didn't want to run the risk of becoming addicted to pills in the hopes of easing the pain. Pain killers always carried with them the promise of side effects, and the possibility of other problems worsening or developing as a result of them. And the possibility of becoming addicted scared me. It would be too easy to throw a bottle of pills in my purse and run off to the girls' play group or dance class or the park, taking pills all the while. And pills were socially acceptable, provoking only sympathy. But it seemed likely I'd get out of control with them—that if they helped the pain as was intended, I'd rely on them. I didn't want to lose sight of my ultimate goal. To become healthy, to repair my body, not to become accustomed to it functioning improperly.

I grew tired of doctors—the visits, their bills, their disagreement on a diagnosis and their general inability to alleviate the pain.

What could I do, I wondered, that maybe the doctors hadn't thought of? Megadoses of vitamins (to supplement my already healthy diet)? Exercise? Not much of a plan of action, I thought, but considering my lack of options I had nothing to lose.

One of the most consistent theories expressed to me was that scar tissue had formed and was now strangling other nerves as well as the one originally injured. "It's like a dam," Dr. Christian had told me, "causing circulatory problems. The blood wells up, can't get through, the cramping increases."

Well, I'll burst the dam, I thought, if I create enough pressure.

Andrew had always loved running, and did so frequently with my brother. Andrew had been a star on our high school track and cross country teams when I met him. "We'll run," he said, thrilled at my optimism and the possibility of not throwing money away on a weekly basis at the doctor's office.

We began running at Pierce College, a local community school. We'd take the girls over with their bikes, and we'd run while they rode along beside us laughing. We were all thrilled at regaining some sense of family. The pain was unbelievable and, even scarier, was increasing. But after nearly two years of hell, I was determined to break up the scar tissue. So I ran.

January 1984, one year eight months after the injection: Sheila, a close and unceasingly supportive friend, called to tell me about the U.C.L.A. Pain Clinic. Sheila was incredible. The mother of four beautiful girls, all under 8, she was full of energy and enthusiasm and had a gift for life.

"Listen Kath," she coaxed me, ever so gently, "I know you're tired of doctors but aren't you more tired of pain? It's a cycle Kathy. And you've got to break it. Give U.C.L.A. a call and see if they can help."

I was convinced in those days that no one understood what I was going through. But her balance of concern and compassion and the example she set in herself inspired me. "I'll do it," I said feeling a tiny surge of adrenaline. "I'll call one more doctor." Hope springs eternal, I thought as I called U.C.L.A.

During this phone call, I was informed that I was not simply making one more doctor's appointment. I was applying as a "candidate for medical treatment at U.C.L.A. Pain Management Center." I would need a doctor's recommendation, complete medical records, extensive paperwork and current insurance coverage information, as well as a battery of psychological tests.

"If all goes well, Mrs. Waddick, you could be accepted here for treatment within ninety days," the voice on the other end of the line gushed optimistically.

How wonderful, I thought, drained already.

Neil, thinking it was a great idea, had a neurologist I had previously seen submit my medical records and a letter requesting treatment for me.

Meanwhile, Neil notified me, it was time for my arbitration. An arbitration would be non-binding, but they frequently led to settlements. Anyway, it was required. "The courts are crowded," he told me. "Arbitrations are mandatory so as not to waste time and taxpayers money. As for you," he said, "you have enough problems. Settling the case would be good all around."

Arbitration

The arbitration was held at a local law school. A retired judge was assigned as arbitrator. A look of surprise appeared on Neil's face when he saw the nurse who had given me the injection, and he began hurriedly shuffling through some files. "My God Kathy," he said, "look at this," and handed me a copy of a deposition I'd given previously.

"Yeah, so?"

"Look at your description of Nurse Racine," he said excitedly. "And look at her," he said pointing to the nurse. "Your recall is remarkable Kathy."

Neil began to question Nurse Racine. How many children did she have? All boys? Did she ski? She had four children she said, all boys, and yes, she skied.

The defense attorney objected that this line of questioning was irrelevant. The arbitrator agreed.

"Your Honor, I'm trying to lay a foundation," Neil said. "I would like to read from a deposition Kathleen took previously, her description of Nurse Racine, and of a conversation they had in the emergency room."

"No," the arbitrator said. "I know perfectly well what the nurse looks like, and any conversation they might have had is irrelevant."

"But Kathleen's power of recall is not," Neil said.

Especially my recall of Nurse Racine saying on the night of the injection that she was working three jobs and hadn't slept in 72 hours, I thought.

"Irrelevant," said the arbitrator. "Move on."

Daisy Racine, the nurse, was wearing shorts, a tube top, a big pink bow on her ponytail and a charm bracelet. She was nervous and giggled through Neil's questioning. She stated that she had no memory of me at all but that she must have administered the injection since "I see my signature here," she said holding up for the judge a slip of paper from my hospital file.

"Are there any instances Nurse Racine," Neil asked, "when one should be careful in administering an injection of Phenergan?" I thought this question absurd, assuming she would state she was always careful when administering any medication. She giggled uneasily and said she didn't know.

The defense had obtained from Dr. Alexander (Marcus Welby) a letter written on their behalf, by him. In it he stated that I'd never complained of pain on the left side of my body, but instead had some vague complaints—nausea, fatigue—the sort of complaints you often see in a mother with young children. And that I'd complained of pain in my *right* leg, saying that my right leg "felt shorter than my left."

Neil, after looking at his copy of Dr. Alexander's file on me, at this point introduced Dr. Alexander's notes on my first visit to see him. "Chief complaint—pain and tenderness" on my "*left*."

Why would Dr. Alexander have written that letter? I wondered.

I remembered Dr. Alexander asking me repeatedly if I didn't have any other complaints, he always looked for alternative reasons for my pain, even minor complaints, he'd say, "as long as you're here."

Neil countered the defense's focus on the pain on the right side. "If Kathleen has an area of extreme sensitivity, it is no surprise that she would shift her body, to guard that area. As a result of this her body might come out of alignment, resulting in pain on the right. I don't know. But I do know," he said, "that it states here that Kathleen's chief complaint to Dr. Alexander was pain on the left. And that she continued to complain of pain on the left throughout her visits to him."

The single most infuriating and eye opening piece of information I was afforded at the arbitration was that it stated right there in my hospital file that I'd been given the injection on the left.

I thought back on my conversation with Dr. Boxer, the chief of staff of the emergency room. I thought about how we'd disagreed about where I'd been given the injection. "I have your file right here Mrs. Waddick and our records clearly indicate the injection was given on the right."

What did this mean? Had he the records in his hand as he'd said, but lied to me hoping I'd go away—or had he never checked my file, not caring whether there had been negligence? Had he just intended to protect the hospital's reputation and insurance rates at whatever cost? How naive I'd been. I'd assumed he would want to know if any of his staff had been careless, and I certainly never thought a doctor would lie.

The defense retained for the arbitration an "expert witness," a neurosurgeon who carried with him "some of his published writings," to which he referred frequently. He was in his sixties, well dressed, self assured and to me unintelligible.

We broke for lunch shortly after the neurosurgeon's testimony. Andrew, Neil and I went to a local coffee shop. I was disheartened, finding their neurosurgeon's testimony intimidating.

"I didn't understand a word he said," Andrew agreed, shaking his head.

"Neither did I," Neil concurred. "I think he's a pompous academic. But he's testifying."

Neil was right. I had no doctor testifying for me. They not only had the neurosurgeon, but they had the letter from one of my own doctors, Dr. Alexander. One willing to fabricate and the other paid to obfuscate.

At the close of the proceeding, the arbitrator said that he found the case straightforward and he had reached a decision. "You'll receive the results in a month or so," he said.

A month! A month that felt like a decade.

At last Neil called. The arbitrator recommended compensation to me of $33,000. After medical bills (and I would have to reimburse the insurance company for the portions of the bills they had covered), Neil's share and the unknown state of my health, this struck me as not just low, but unacceptable.

"It is low, Kath," Neil said. "But keep in mind they had an expert witness present *and* Dr. Alexander's false testimonial letter. Despite this, the arbitrator said he found this case straightforward and ruled in your favor. The award was just low. Arbitration awards are generally low."

All the same, I'd won the arbitration.

A feather in my cap, I thought.

April 1984: I began to wear thin. While running helped emotionally—I felt better, stronger, clearer—physically, it was agonizing. I had to beat it, I told myself. The entire time I was running, I envisioned the dam bursting and the pain disappearing. Meanwhile, the pain was building. The area where I'd had the injection seemed to hold every conceivable type of pain, all at the same time.

One night about 9 p.m., with Andrew at home and the girls tucked in bed, I poured myself a glass of wine, and then another. I needed to unwind, to fall asleep, I told myself. It helped, and I followed suit the next night and the next. I drank wine, or beer, or liqueurs we'd had around the house for years untouched—Christmas gifts, etc.

This shocked Andrew. "What are you doing, Kathy?"

"Dulling the pain so I can fall asleep, Andrew. As soon as the running starts to help, or the doctors come up with something, I'll stop. Anyway, you're here and the girls are asleep. It's not like I'd ever throw a bottle of alcohol in my purse to drink during the day like I could pills. And it's temporary," I said. "Just until something changes."

Commitment

"Almost all our faults are more pardonable than the methods we think up to hide them."

—Francois de La Rouchefoucald

June 1984: I was notified of an appointment date at U.C.L.A. to take the MMPI as part of the initial screening for treatment at the Pain Clinic. The Minnesota Multiphasic Personality Inventory was a psychological test consisting of some 565 questions.

The day of the MMPI, I was directed to a small room, crowded with desks, a chalkboard, and little else. A tall, thin woman entered the room and instructed us not to deliberate over, or attempt to analyze any of the questions. But to answer each one, "even though some of the questions may seem a bit strange." She then left the room and with no other medical personnel present we all dutifully began to complete the questionnaire. By the end of the first page I was laughing. Aloud. It struck me that I rarely laughed anymore and that I should probably request a copy of the test, to take home, for amusement sake.

Then an uncomfortable thought crossed my mind. I was the only one laughing. Here I was in a crowded, depressing room packed with people reading strange, ridiculous true/false statements such as:

> *My soul sometimes leaves my body.*
> *I am a special agent of God.*
> *I used to like drop the handkerchief.*
> *I think Lincoln was greater than Washington.*
> *I like repairing a door latch.*
> *I like tall women.*

Did they really believe they would get to know me better by asking me these things? And better yet, was I to believe this would enable them to help the pain? However, it had been made clear that this was a *mandatory* step to treatment at the pain clinic. Stupid or not, I needed to complete this questionnaire.

How do I answer? I wondered as I tried to think about tall women. Neither true nor false struck me as a desirable answer. True, I like tall women. Tall women as opposed to what? And in what way are we talking about me liking them? False. Does that mean I do not like tall women, but I like short women? Or does that mean I do not like women? Does that mean I do not like myself? I chose true, uncomfortably.

> *I do not like to see women smoke. True/False*

Here we go again, I thought. I'm not fond of smoking, but I felt uncomfortable singling out women. I chose true again however because it came closest to the truth.

Then I came to the physical true/false questions.

I have little or no trouble with my muscles twitching and jumping.

> *I have few or no pains.*
> *I have numbness in one or more regions of my skin.*
> *My skin seems to be unusually sensitive to touch.*
> *I do not dread seeing a doctor about sickness or injury.*

I wondered whether the computer that translated my answers into a psychological profile would know my recent physical history.

> *Evil spirits possess me at times.*
> *I see things or animals or people around me that others do not see.*

Oh good, I thought, we're getting back into comfortable territory where I can easily, truthfully answer a question without having an argument with myself. But how about,

> *Sometimes I feel as if I must injure either myself or someone else.*

They probably wouldn't ask this question if they didn't think it was a possibility. What if someone here does often feel like harming others? We're all admittedly under stress. What if reading this gets him thinking, inspires him? What if the someone he chooses to harm is me?

My new objective was to get the hell out of there. I thought back on school tests when teachers had uttered the magic words, "Class, when you are done with your test, done being each question answered, you may go home." I quickened my pace.

The woman directly in front of me was elderly and unable to read the questions herself. Her husband read them to her, berated her for thinking them over for too long, and argued with her answers. The woman next to me, according to her mother, was "in far too much pain to read;" therefore her mother read the questions to her, finding it necessary to repeat each one several times, as her daughter was also "in far too much pain to think." Also in the room was a man unable to read English, thus requiring an interpreter, and an elderly woman in a hospital bed, oblivious to all but her own seemingly agonizing pain. A young couple accompanying her filled out her MMPI, involving themselves in somewhat lengthy discussions over each question, with the woman in the hospital bed crying all the while. Every so often the tall, thin woman would re-enter the room and remind all of us there should be no talking. "We wouldn't want to distract our neighbors, now would we?"

"My sex life is satisfactory," read the elderly man in front of me to his wife.

"Yes," she said immediately, not taking her customary several minutes to mull the question over in her mind.

Seeming quite taken aback he argued with her, "What sex life? We haven't had sex in years!"

"And that's why I'm so satisfied," she said sweetly.

On the follow up visit, after the MMPI, but before a treatment plan had been selected, Dr. Elliot, the pain clinic's neurologist, examined me. She performed a physical examination and talked with me for awhile.

Did that clicking in my jaw bother me? she asked.

I had never thought about the clicking. I laughed. "That's the least of my troubles."

"O.K.," she said lightly, moving on to a slew of questions. Did the intensity of the pain vary? Could I see a pattern? What helped? What didn't? Was my family supportive?

"Can you help?" I almost whispered.

"I think so," she said.

"You do?" I asked, astonished, my heart racing.

"Frankly, Kathleen," she said, "I think that you are the most over diagnosed and undertreated patient I have ever seen. I believe there are a variety of therapies we can try; I'd like to start with the least invasive. To be honest though, your depression and your drinking concern me more than anything."

To be honest, I thought, I don't care what concerns you more than anything. I care that you believe there are a variety of therapies we can try. I care that you have hope. Because now I can hope too, but—"In this pain Dr. Elliot it would be hard for me not to be depressed. As far as the drinking, that stemmed from the pain and hopelessness."

Dr. Elliot didn't look up as I spoke, but continued writing. "It's time for you to see Dr. Millston now Kathleen. She's our staff psychologist. She'll go over your MMPI test results with you."

Dr. Millston, I soon found, was the one who had given us the MMPI. Now, alone with her in her office, she went on and on as to what my MMPI test results reflected. "Your test results, Kathleen, indicate you have markedly feminine interests, that your level of stress is quite high at this time, and that you are severely depressed. Furthermore ..."

I couldn't follow her. I was exhausted and in pain and my mind kept wandering. I was excited by Dr. Elliot's optimism but I was scared. I didn't want to get my hopes up. They'd been dashed too many times.

"Mrs. Waddick," she said, "are you listening to me?"

Dr. Millston, I thought, I'm trying to listen to you. But my mind is wandering, my thoughts racing. I'm certain it's in my best interest to listen to you, but I don't know what you're talking about.

"Mrs. Waddick, Dr. Elliot and I are gravely concerned with your mood... and your drinking."

"Dr. Millston," I said, "in my worst nightmares, I've never imagined a person could live in as much pain, every day, all day, as I have been in for nearly two-and-a-half years. I can't describe this pain, I can't deal with this pain, and as arrogant as it sounds, I don't believe for a minute you could either. One doctor after another has been confused by it, and suggested that I needed to 'accept' it, to learn to 'live' with it, or perhaps that it simply didn't exist. My depression is not something to concern yourself with. My pain is. When the pain is alleviated my depression will lift. As for my drinking—first off, I've only been drinking alcohol for four months. Second, alcohol has been a by-product of the pain. No pain—no alcohol—no depression."

"Mrs. Waddick," she said smiling stiffly, "I'm here to help you. My primary concern is your welfare. Your depression is serious, and we must take the necessary steps to clear it up."

Here we go again, I thought. Of course I wanted my depression "cleared up" and yes I agreed, drinking was not a good thing. But they were by-products. Why was everyone more concerned with them?

"Mrs. Waddick, in view of the severity of your depression, I'd like you to see Dr. Marks, our staff psychiatrist. Would you be willing to do this?" she asked in a tone most people reserved for small children.

My thoughts were a jumble. I tried to sort them out. Dr. Elliot had said I was both over diagnosed and undertreated, and that there were a variety of therapies we could try.

I'd taken their nutty test... *I am a special agent of God. My soul sometimes leaves my body. I see things or animals or people around me that others do not see.* I had waited months for word that I would be accepted as a possible "candidate" for treatment at the pain clinic. I had been in pain now for a long time. My home life was disintegrating, and I was worn down, not just physically but emotionally as well.

And rather than starting one of the "variety of therapies" they could try they wanted me to see a *psychiatrist*?

This did not sit well with me. I had enough anxiety about the medical profession. I was tired of painful exams that turned up nothing. I was tired of doctors that charged me but couldn't help. Over two years later, I still found it incomprehensible that Dr. Alexander had treated me over a three month period, then said that he thought it was emotional *and* written a letter to be used against me in court.

I was bothered that Dr. Shein had cited early disc disease, suggesting that I'd been experiencing pain for quite some time, but that I just hadn't been "aware of it." And that Dr. Daniels had seemed more concerned with the possibility of a negative reaction from colleagues and the A.M.A. than with my problems. And after Dr. Daniels, there had been Dr. Christian, and then a slew of others, prescribing pills, rest—how was I to achieve that!—and a dozen different diagnoses.

Most promised they could help early on, and each time it hurt more when they couldn't. I was afraid to get my hopes up one more time. And I was still confused as to why, after a lengthy admission procedure, I'd have to spend so much time taking peculiar tests and speaking with their staff psychologist. And now a psychiatrist?

Dr. Marks struck me as intelligent and focused. I didn't get the feeling that the entire time I was talking to him, he was choosing his next words and just waiting for me to pause. He seemed to respond to me. Not a clinical impression of me, but me. I liked him. Enormously. One would never have thought so however. I was cold, sarcastic and abrasive. I wanted to get on with it! I wanted the pain addressed. All my problems it seemed had begun with the medical profession and now I felt no one was taking any responsibility for the negligence. And in addition to not taking any responsibility—some people were lying.

And so here I was, on the one hand wanting to like Dr. Marks, to open up to him, to tell him I needed help. But I didn't want to be vulnerable, especially with one of "them." Nor did I want to waste time with a *psychiatrist.*

I answered his gentle inquiries with "What's it to you?" and "Why do you ask doctor? Do you want to help me? Well please don't! I'd say the whole damn medical profession has done enough for me already, wouldn't you?" Dr. Marks made it clear that he understood my anger and my difficulty in trusting him, but that he had no desire to be my punching bag. He said that the stress I'd been under must be overwhelming.

He asked if nearly two and a half years of interrupted sleep, totaling ridiculously small amounts daily, two and a half years of constant pain, an injury remaining undiagnosed, and doctors turning their backs on their ethical and moral obligations wasn't more than I could deal with alone?

I wanted to say that it was and that I couldn't believe that he understood, and that I didn't want to feel so alone, to be so alone, but that would have meant that I would have had to trust him. And although my gut told me that I could trust him, intellectually I thought I'd be nuts to wear my heart on my sleeve, and to hope much good could come from him.

So I said tauntingly, "So tell me doc, are you really so different?"

"You're very angry Kathleen."

"With reason to be," I shot back.

"You're so unhappy Kathleen," he said leaning towards me. "Do you ever think of committing suicide?"

"Every day," I said disgusted by this ridiculous question. I'd like to meet a person experiencing this much pain, I thought, that never thinks of suicide. I quickly looked away, not wanting him to sense my fear and desperation.

"How do you imagine taking your life?" he asked.

"Well," I paused, already exhausted by the conversation, "on the way here today I had all I could do not to drive off the freeway. It seemed so promising. No more pain, eternal sleep. And at night I have an overwhelming urge to stab myself. I feel a constant stabbing where I had the injection anyway so I think sheesh, with one good stab I wouldn't feel any more. I'd just be at peace. And other times I think an overdose would be the simplest, and oh, what the fuck do I know?" I said, my voice trailing off.

"And what of your dreams Kathleen, do you dream?"

"I have nightmares, the same two every night."

"What are they?" he asked seeming quite interested.

I sighed. "Well, one is that Andrew goes with me to see a doctor. We enter the office and the doctor is seated behind an enormous desk. He motions for us to sit down, and we do. The doctor says that after reviewing my records it's clear to him that there is only one treatment he can recommend. 'And what's that?' I ask, feeling excited and hopeful. 'For you to have an injection on your right, as you've had on your left. That will relieve that uncomfortable 'different' feeling you experience Mrs. Waddick.' I stand up, appalled, horrified, wanting to leave, but Andrew remains seated, actually listening to this. I look at Andrew in disbelief, and when I look back at the doctor I can no longer understand anything he is saying to me. His mouth is moving but I can't make heads or tails of anything he is saying. He speaks quickly and seemingly in a foreign language. And yet Andrew is conversing with him and I become terrified. Just when I can't stand any more of it, Andrew stands up, takes my hand and squeezes it, and tells me that everything is going to be O.K. He then leads me by the hand out the door and down a long corridor, and when we reach the end a door seemingly opens of its own accord and Andrew gently nudges me in. Sensing Andrew recoiling, I turn to him. Backing away, looking grief stricken he says pleading, 'I had to do it Kathy. I *had* to do it.' And I realize he's just committed me to a psychiatric ward. I try to shriek, but no sound escapes. Then I wake up. As for the other nightmare —"

"Kathleen," Dr. Marks interrupted. "You are not crazy," he said emphatically. "But you are sick. You need help. Since the injection, you have been in continual pain, sleeping improperly, probably eating improperly. You are suffering from a chemical imbalance," he said, "and I think we can help. To what degree I am not sure, but you are very depressed. You scare me. Now I'd like to check you into the hospital for awhile."

"To the neurology ward?" I asked.

"To the psychiatric ward," he said haltingly.

"Who the fuck are you?" I exploded. "You think I'm nuts. You all think I'm nuts. You just keep stringing me along, taking my money all the while. I don't want to be in a psychiatric ward. I am not crazy. You all give me tests and fill your files with them and talk about my 'personality profile.' You have me come here but you don't even believe I'm in pain, or perhaps I should say physical pain. Gee, you don't seem like a person in chronic pain, everyone says. Well, I seem just like a person in chronic pain. But I'm an individual—and people in chronic pain respond *individually*. We do not respond 'accordingly.' We are not cattle! What is it with you people?"

"Kathleen, you're very angry and you're very depressed. Let me call your husband to come and get you."

"No," I said curtly, "I'm fine."

"Well, then how about your mother," he asked. "Or a friend."

"No," I repeated, "Nobody!" I had grown terrified at the thought of ending up all alone. I was headed that way, I was sure. I'd grown tired and sick and horrible to be around. I wanted to say, there's no one to call! Do you know how inconvenienced my friends and family have been? I'm afraid they're getting sick of me. My problem has become theirs. I can't call them because I'm afraid it will be the straw that breaks the camel's back and then I'll be all alone.

Glancing at his watch, Dr. Marks jumped up. "Excuse me for one minute Kathleen. I just realized I need to arrange to have some tests run on you today, before it's too late."

"What kind of tests?" I asked.

"A kidney test for one," he said opening the door.

"What's the matter?" I asked full of sarcasm. "Afraid I damaged my kidneys drinking all that alcohol?"

"As a matter of fact I am," he said softly.

I felt unsettled. He cares, I thought, as I sat waiting for him. But why was he concerned with a kidney test? Why wasn't he concerned with alleviating the pain? How could my kidneys warrant this interest after only four months of drinking? I'd been in continual pain for two and a half years, why wasn't that the focus?

A couple of minutes later he returned with two hospital guards in uniform. I panicked. "Kathleen —" Dr. Marks started.

"You can't do this," I hissed, gripping the sides of the chair. "You can't put me in the hospital, you can't..."

"Kathleen, I can. I didn't want to," he said looking pained. "I thought about it, but you left me no choice."

"I trusted you," I whispered.

"Kathleen, you refused to admit yourself, or to involve your husband, or your mother."

Refuse to involve my husband or my mother I thought? They were so involved I couldn't stand it. The pain wasn't only ruining my life but theirs and my daughters as well.

"You desperately need help Kathleen, and you're too sick to see it."

Too sick to see it? I was begging for help the way I saw it.

The guards made a small step toward me. I stood up quickly. With my sanity in question I felt compelled to react "normally."

The walk to NPI, the Neuro Psychiatric Institute, was a long one and the guards walked close on either side of me. Dr. Marks came too.

"Dr. Marks," I said quietly, "don't do this. It won't help."

"I'll visit you every day Kathleen," he said.

Visit me? I thought. That's great. Lock me up, but promise to visit me.

Passersby in the hall stared at me. I felt embarrassed, naked.

Having delivered me to NPI, Dr. Marks assured me he'd be in touch soon and once again that he would visit. I was petrified. The very thought of a psychiatric ward sent chills up my spine and made my head pound. I didn't know what to do and I decided anything I did to get out of there was justifiable. I couldn't stay there, locked up.

After a long wait, a young doctor came in. It would be his task to evaluate me he said. "What is going on with you?" he asked. Was I really so depressed? Should Dr. Marks really be so concerned, he asked? I didn't look it to him, he said.

"Well, Dr. Bellamy," I said carefully choosing each word, "I assume Dr. Marks mentioned to you my chronic pain problem. He asked if I ever had thoughts of suicide. I said I do. I imagine anyone would, I said."

"That's it?" he asked, surprised.

"That's it," I answered, smiling and trying to appear amused. "To be honest with you, Dr. Bellamy, I appreciate his concern. But you see tomorrow I'm having a bridal shower for my future sister in law.

I'd hate to cancel it. If you want me to admit myself as soon as it's over, I will. I promise! But I can't ruin Joy's wedding shower!"

"Well Mrs. Waddick," he said, standing up "you seem fine to me. We're crowded enough on the wards at this time, and no one planning a wedding shower is suicidal enough to be locked up. But I can't let you leave here alone. Can you understand that?"

"Sure I do," I said smiling, "you can give my mom a call if you want. She works close by."

After phoning my mom he wrote me three prescriptions and asked me to wait in the reception area for her. Tired of being inside, I slipped past the receptionist who was to "keep an eye" on me, and waited on the steps outside.

My mom worked nearby and yet it was quite a while before she arrived. She'd become upset, she said, when the doctor had called telling her they'd considered committing me but would release me to her providing she didn't allow me to drive, or to remain alone. So upset, she'd gotten lost three times on the way to get me.

"Why are you out here alone?" she asked. She looked pale, concerned, out of breath. "The doctor said they'd be keeping an eye on you. Come on," she said, taking my arm.

"My car's not over here," I said. "It's in the parking structure."

"Well you come home with me, honey," she said. "We'll get your car later."

"Don't be ridiculous," I told her. "I'm fine. Why should I leave my car here?"

I couldn't believe my own mother was going to begin letting the emotional aspects of my problem overshadow the physical.

"Honey, they asked me not to let you drive," she said looking uncomfortable. "I just never had any idea how depressed you are. I would have never guessed there was cause to be so concerned."

"I'm fine," I said again, "surely you can see that."

"I'm just worried," she said. "I don't want anything to happen to you."

"Look at me, I'm fine!" I said hugging her. "I'll see you at home, I promise!"

Twenty minutes later, on the freeway, I had no idea where I was. Freeway signs seemed familiar, but I couldn't remember where to exit, or where I lived. I pulled off the freeway and parked. I sat there confused, feeling overcome by exhaustion. Then I began to rummage through my purse. Checkbook in hand, I pulled into a nearby gas station and asked where the address on the checks was.

When I arrived home my mother was there waiting for me. "See why I don't like freeways," she said, "I made it here quicker than you, over Sepulveda."

"Another main area of complaint is 'depression.' However, the patient tells me that 'I didn't think I had it,' indicating that depression as a chemical diagnosis was not something that she recognized."

— *Dr. Wilhelm Payne, defense psychiatrist*

I never allowed myself to be alone with the girls after this, concerned for their safety, as it was clear my mind was slipping. My brother was due to be married in late August. I didn't want to ruin his wedding, but I didn't know how long I could hold on.

And so about two weeks later, the day after the wedding, I called Dr. Marks. His exchange said they would beep him. It was well after office hours but he returned my call quickly.

"Did I get you in trouble?" I asked him, referring to my release after his attempt to commit me.

"Not at all," he said gently.

"I'm sorry Dr. Marks, but I had to get out of there."

"Kathleen, I've been worried about you. How are you doing?"

"Not good," I said. "I need help."

"You need," he said, "to be in the hospital."

"But not in a psych ward," I said, feeling a chill. Couldn't he admit me to the neurology ward? He'd look into it he said, and call me the next morning.

He'd just spoken with Dr. Elliot, Dr. Marks said the next morning. And she was far too concerned with my mood to want to begin treating my pain, therefore the neurology ward was out. The anger began to well up inside of me. She wanted my depression cleared up first, he continued, which she felt was just too intense for the "invasive" therapies required to begin treating me. There was no mention of the non-invasive therapies Dr. Elliot had excited me with during her examination.

"Well, I don't want to go in a psych ward. If I return to the pain clinic for outpatient treatment will there be a repeat attempt to commit me?"

"Kathleen, I can't answer that."

"But that's stupid," I said. "I won't return if that's the case, and then I won't be helped at all. Perhaps in-hospital treatment would move quicker but outpatient treatment would certainly be better than none."

"Kathleen, it's not the speed of the therapy we want you in the hospital for. I believe you need to be somewhere safe right now. You are sick. You have a chemical imbalance and it is critical you receive treatment."

"Dr. Marks," I said irritated, "I've never heard of a chemical imbalance, and neither has anyone else I've mentioned it to since the last time I saw you. How do I know you don't just think I'm nuts?"

"Well, I guess you don't know," he said. "But maybe you need to take the chance and trust me. What alternative do you have anyway? We can clear up your depression, your poor sleeping, and down the road begin treatments for your pain. If *you* admit yourself into NPI, you'll have more responsibility, more freedom. You'll be taking an active part in your treatment program. We won't be doing this to you but with you."

I'll think about it, I said, feeling cornered.

I went to see Neil, both wondering what a psychiatric hospitalization would do to my case, and wanting advice. I was shaky, forgetful, anxious. I walked into his office, he kept writing, obviously busy. I told Neil as briefly as I could about the whole catch-22—that my depression would have to be treated before they would treat the pain that caused it. A psychiatric ward for me? I asked, on the verge of crying.

"You cut your hair," he said looking at me for the first time. "I liked it better long."

Had he been listening? Did he realize the importance of what I was saying?

"This isn't going to help your case Kath, and it's definitely going to complicate it. But if you have to do it, then go ahead," he said standing up, walking me to the door.

I walked out onto Wilshire Boulevard, a jumble of emotions more complicated than before I'd seen Neil. I was suicidal; I knew that.

"Well then that's a good place for you," Neil had said when I told him this.

Supposedly my sanity wasn't in question. I was suffering from a chemical imbalance due to stress, Dr. Marks said. And yet I'd never heard of a chemical imbalance. Dr. Marks' words, "What alternative do you have anyway?" kept going through my mind.

When I arrived home visibly shaken Andrew insisted we all go to a neighborhood park.

"Take the girls down the slide Kath," Andrew said as we pulled up. "You used to love that." Sensing my hesitation, he continued, "Go on. It would do you good."

Tears streamed down my face. "Do me good? Do you have any idea what that would feel like on the area where I had the injection?"

"No Kathy, I don't," he said pausing. "I don't know *much* about you anymore, and I wonder what life holds for us. I just keep on working, hoping that one day I'll come home and the old Kathy will meet me at the door."

"Don't you think I wish the same Andrew? Don't you think I miss feeling good? Do you think I like all of this? And what it's doing to the girls? And to you and my mom?"

"Well, what are you going to do?" he asked wearily.

"It used to be what are *we* going to do Andrew. Is that what it's come to? I'm on my own?"

"You're not on your own Kathy. I'm here, aren't I? But I'm burned out. I don't have any ideas. I just know I can't live like this."

"That makes two of us," I said, feeling the world closing in on me.

I looked over at the girls playing quietly, watching me out of the corner of their eyes. Two little girls, three and five, whose childhood was crumbling because of me. I didn't want to ruin everyone's life along with mine. I didn't know what to do, but I didn't see myself as crazy enough to be locked up in a psychiatric ward.

Didn't just the fact that I was here trying to reason all this through cancel me out as a candidate for a nut house?

"A phenomenon that a number of people have noted while in deep depression is the sense of being accompanied by a second self—a wraithlike observer who, not sharing the dementia of his double, is able to watch with dispassionate curiosity as his companion struggles against the oncoming disaster, or decides to embrace it."

—William Styron

In the middle of the night, I woke up with an intense desire to kill myself. The area where I had the injection felt on fire and was cramping, as well as the continual stabbing, shooting pains. One good stab with a kitchen knife, I thought, and I would never have to feel this again.

This was not a new thought, but I'd never felt so intense about it before. It was as though there were now two people inside my head. One person saying kindly, gently, in the tone you would urge your baby to take his first step, "Go ahead Kathy. Kill yourself. It will be wonderful. Eternal peace. No more pain. Not just for you but for the girls as well. For everyone really." The other voice was angry, and talking at the same time, "Don't be crazy. Killing yourself wouldn't help the girls live a more peaceful life. It would be taking *your* chronic pain and passing it on to them. The pain of having you kill yourself would never, never go away."

I found myself in the kitchen with a knife in my hand. Go ahead, do it, I found myself repeating. I was dripping with sweat and shaking from head to toe. "Do it!" I was telling myself. "Don't be crazy!" I was telling myself. I ran into our bedroom, knife in hand.

"Andrew, I need you. Wake up, I'm afraid I'm going to kill myself."

"You're not going to kill yourself," he said rubbing his eyes, barely awake.

"Andrew, listen, something is wrong with me. I feel strange. I feel excited that it's almost all over for me, and horror at what I'm going to do."

"You're not going to do that, Kathy. Please, I have to get up for work at five. I need to get some sleep."

"Andrew," I said pleading, short of breath, "Don't go to sleep. I need you."

"And I need some sleep Kathy. Let's talk tomorrow, okay?"

Shaking and sweating profusely, I sat in the living room for the rest of the night arguing with myself.

In the morning, I phoned Dr. Marks. "I need help. I'm willing to sign myself in. I'm willing to commit myself." The words came tumbling out.

"O.K., good, Kathleen," Dr. Marks said sighing. "I know we can help you."

"But how long do you think I'd need to stay?" I asked.

"About a week, Kathleen."

"A week? People get out of the hospital in a day or two after surgery. A week is a long time to be in the hospital."

"Not considering the severity of your depression. A week should give us just enough time to get a handle on things."

A week.

And so the cleaning and shopping and laundry and lists began. I kept trying to view admitting myself to a psychiatric ward as a positive, as a beginning. But I was terrified. There I would be with a bunch of nuts. Didn't that make me nuts? Weren't these people dangerous? It had been made clear to me I couldn't have a private room. I'd have to share a room! With whom? I worried.

Just the fact that I was capable of filling the house with groceries and preparing lists for taking care of the girls made me wonder how I could be crazy enough to need hospitalization. But the possibility of a reenactment of the previous night's horror was too terrifying a thought. The day, the sunshine and the girls laughter brought me back, just barely, into contact with the real world. The night carried terror.

As I was packing, Acasia and Amanda asked, "Will they fix you mommy? Will you be home soon? Why don't they come here and fix you? Why can't we go with you? Will you miss us?"

And when I was unable to respond quickly, Amanda's face tightened and she shook me, "Do you *want* to go mommy?"

Psych Ward

"The most important kind of tolerance is tolerance of the individual by society and the state."

—Albert Einstein

August 30, 1984: That first day checking into the psychiatric ward, the nurse took my make-up, my mirror, my hair blower and my razor away and labeled them. I would need to check these items in and out as I needed them, and there would be a twenty minute time limit, she said. After all, I could hurt myself with these things. With my makeup case? I asked, dumfounded. You could break it, she said staring me straight in the face, and harm yourself with a jagged edge.

I was instructed that for the first 24 hours I should "save" all my urine in a labeled container, "turning it in" routinely to the nursing station. The container was large, transparent, conspicuous and I was embarrassed. The first time I approached the nursing station with the container I knocked on the door to the station that entered from the women's hall, rather than going out to the shared front hall which was both co-ed and busy. The nurse indicated that I would have to go to the front hall with it. There were about five or six other patients ahead of me.

And so I stood there, in line, with a container full of urine, waiting my turn.

I was later told the urine had not been for any particular tests pertaining to me, but part of a "study" the university was doing.

What better patient to humiliate than a mentally ill one I thought.

Dr. Jones immediately arranged for me to have brief visits with the girls, in the hall outside of the ward, waiving the standard 3 day screening period, during which patients are not allowed to leave the ward.

"Talk to me, Kathleen," Dr. Jones gently urged.

"There's nothing to say. I wish I was dead."

"You're terribly depressed, Kathleen. But you wait and see. We'll get a handle on this depression," he said hopefully. "And then you'll see how much you have to live for."

"Dr. Jones," I said flatly, "I am removed from my one reason to remain alive — Acasia and Amanda. The world's closing in around me and I just want to be dead."

"But you'd never see Acasia and Amanda again, Kathleen."

"They'd be better off."

"Better off? Kathleen, how could two little girls be better off without their mother?"

"Look at me."

"Kathleen, that's depression talking. You won't always feel this way. We'll get your depression cleared up, and you'll remember why you're alive. You'll laugh again."

"Laugh?" I repeated incredulously. Had I ever laughed, I wondered? My whole sense of time was gone. I couldn't remember when things had ever been any different. I just knew that I hated myself, and that I had become a horrible burden to everyone I loved.

"Kathleen, listen to me. I know how you're feeling. But you are suffering from a chemical imbalance. You're not responsible for the onset of your depression, and you're incapable of clearing it up. All you know is you want to be dead. Not out of weakness, but because you are sick. You've been through hell. We can help you. But you need to trust me."

"I trust you," I said truthfully. "It's just that there's nothing you can do."

"That's the point Kathleen. I don't agree. I think there is a great deal we can do. You need to just sit back and do nothing for a little while. Take a break. You be the passenger. Let me do the work. You be the patient."

But as the patient I felt like a piece of meat. We were treated much of the time like cattle. Sick cattle. Lined up for our meals, our "meds", blood tests. Next, next, next.

Treatments at the pain clinic did not begin. The pain clinic, I was told, was "following" my progress and did not yet feel "comfortable" with it. I didn't feel "comfortable" locked up and not having the chronic pain addressed.

I missed the girls terribly.

"When can I go home?" I asked Dr. Jones, toward the end of the first week.

"We think we might have your depression cleared up within a month," he said slowly.

"A month?" I nearly shrieked. "Dr. Marks said it would take about a week."

"I don't think anyone had any idea as to the severity of your depression before now Kathleen."

"Maybe, or maybe they knew I'd be unwilling to commit myself *for a month*!"

"Kathleen, I know a month seems like forever, but we're trying to help you, not deceive you. It took a long time for you to reach this level of depression. We can't clear it up much quicker than thirty days."

"I don't know how you think you can clear it up at all with me being away from the one thing I have to live for. I miss Amanda and Acasia," I said, my voice wavering. I felt like there wasn't enough air. I felt the room spinning. How could I get across how stupid this all was, locking me up with a bunch of nuts, staring at me 24 hours a day, and separating me from the girls. "All this," I said exasperated, "for treatment at the pain clinic. When will treatments begin anyway? I've lost too much time already. And now I'm beginning to lose touch entirely."

"What about Andrew, Kathleen? What kind of future do you imagine the two of you have together?"

No words made themselves available to me. I felt dizzy and hot.

"Do you miss Andrew, Kathleen?"

"Sometimes," I said slowly. My mind began to wander. It dawned on me that what I missed was loving Andrew, and what I felt was a tremendous sense of loss because where there had been love before, now I could only get in touch with an enormous sense of relief at being away from him.

Every time I looked at Andrew, I felt overwhelmed by guilt and frustration. He was the same old Andrew, waiting for the same old Kathleen. And she was gone forever, with no one in her place.

"Kathleen?"

I could hear Dr. Jones talking to me, but there was too much noise and confusion in my head to know what to say to him.

I felt too tired. It all seemed so futile. What was the purpose of all this talking anyway? There was nothing new to say. My past had faded, I could barely remember it. The future seemed inconceivable — and undesirable. I knew only the moment. I was in living hell.

Andrew and I agreed he would visit infrequently. He would work — we needed the money — and spend every non-working minute with the girls. And what we didn't say was, we desperately needed a break from each other.

In one of our last serious discussions, he'd said, "*Are* you crazy Kath? I mean I don't know, you don't seem it. But then that's the problem. You look *fine*. But you keep saying you hurt, and God knows I want to believe you — but then the doctors, they either can't find anything wrong or can't agree on a diagnosis, and any which way you look at it, can't help you. All I know is, I keep working and waiting and praying."

My mother visited frequently, with the girls whenever possible, otherwise alone. She was wonderful to me, telling me affectionate stories about the girls that, although I had a hard time following, I wanted to hear. It took a tremendous amount of the little energy I had to hear about the girls, because it made my heart ache. But I needed to hear as much as I could absorb about Amanda and Acasia. I'd seem to drift in and out of consciousness, and when she would sense she was losing me, she would switch to some lighthearted story about her work as a restaurant hostess. And when I was entirely black, she would sit and hold my hand. I remember wanting to reach out to her. But I was numb. I remember thoughts I was unable to express, and I remember feeling that I didn't really exist. That I had already died; that I had become just an observer.

I was charged over $500 a day and required to make my own bed, wash my own clothes, wait in a cafeteria line for bland, over-cooked food, and clear my own dishes. What the hell were they doing with all the money anyway, I wondered. Why could I stay at a world class hotel and be waited on hand and foot for less money?

I felt that if my freedom was taken away, so too should my responsibilities. Standing up was an effort, let alone doing laundry and clearing dishes.

I was angered not only by the complete loss of freedom but the expectation that we would live in that strange place, and go through the motions as though we were at summer camp.

Reluctantly I began settling into hospital routine. Slowly I began to spend time with the other patients. While upon my admission I'd lumped all the other patients together, thinking myself and my situation as entirely unique, and in fact superior, I soon began to see differently.

Our reasons for being hospitalized greatly varied but we shared in that, for whatever reason, we'd lost the ability to cope "out there." And that is why a bond developed between many of us that under different circumstances would have been most unlikely.

We spent a considerable period of time spewing out the various injustices we'd both seen and been a party to. Why, we wondered, was becoming *physically* ill, especially to the point of hospitalization, almost an unquestioned guarantee of receiving flowers and candy and visitors and sympathy. While mental illness brought embarrassment, isolation and anger from supposed loved ones.

"You're doing this to yourself," we'd all heard over and over, "so just stop." Some of us at one time or another had attempted to suggest that heart problems, ulcers, and lung cancer are in some cases "done to ourselves."

"Oh you know what we mean," would be the reply. "Cancer and heart problems are real, physical problems. But you can stop all *this* nonsense any time you want to."

How we wished that was true, and that we could in fact "stop all this nonsense." Immediately.

We used to marvel at how much sicker some of the family members that faithfully visited seemed than the patient they were visiting. I remembered Daisy, the woman who had almost choked me on the day of my admission, saying, "They admitted the wrong one you know."

In my case or hers, I wondered.

Each patient was assigned an activity level from 0 to 5:

0 – Bed restriction
1 – Restricted to the ward
2 – Allowed to leave the ward one on one with medical personnel
3 – Able to leave the ward with a group of patients and a staff member
4 – Able to come and go with another "4" or "5" or friend, staff or family member
5 – Able to come and go as you please while keeping up with appropriate ward activities

As a rule, once admitted, a patient remained a "1" for 72 hours, for observation purposes. You were then able to work your way up or down the scale based on your behavior. Patients with an activity level of 4 or above took evening walks nearly every night, providing we had been good and staff size was at a comfortable level.

During these walks we would frequently be allowed to choose a movie to rent. I had a hard time fathoming that the nursing staff allowed the rental of "One Flew Over the Cuckoo's Nest," "The Big Chill," and a variety of other depressing movies.

"Majority rules," the staff would say, denying responsibility. The majority of us are suicidal, I thought. How about we get some knives?

"Life is a tragedy for those who feel, and a comedy for those who think."

—La Bruyere

I never asked anyone why they were locked up. Reasons for psychiatric hospitalization were far too personal to inquire about — although we did have a few shining stars among us, that wandered the ward saying, "So, what's wrong with you, anyway?" and "So are you one of the ones with a screw loose?" If the same was asked of them, they would laugh and say, "Hah! You thought I was a patient? I'm a plant. I'm paid to keep my eye on *you*."

Some of the patients seemed hopelessly out of touch with reality, and I was certain they would never get better. Others, I could only guess at their reason for hospitalization, through something said in group therapy, or from a visitor, or from the type of medication given, or from their behavior.

Brent, the patient that scared me the day of my admission, "flashed" one day. Calmly, quietly, he pulled down his pants and walked around the day room, exposing himself methodically to each patient. No one had much of a response.

One patient, Nicole, a young girl admitted for anorexia, wasn't on the ward at the time. She returned about an hour later, and Brent, who rarely spoke, approached her. "Nicole," he said deadpan, "you missed something while you were out," and he pulled his pants down once again.

Another patient, Bess, a crusty older woman and an alcoholic, said dryly, "Look Brent, what you got isn't real special. I suggest you keep it to yourself."

Brent was put in restraints and medicated even more heavily than usual, with the nurses citing a recent change in medication as the reason for his "behavior."

Jessica was about 28, intelligent, pretty and always bubbling about her coming wedding. Her fiancé visited daily, and I had no idea why she was there.

One afternoon in the ward bathroom, I heard someone vomiting violently. I immediately alerted the nursing station. Jessica later told me it had been her. She was bulimic, she said, and furious with me for telling on her. Her Activity Level was reduced as a result, and it was a week before she forgave me.

Bob was a quiet, seemingly inoffensive man who showed up on the women's side of the ward one morning, because the men's side was full. Bob frequently wound up in the ladies room staring at us showering. "He's disoriented," the nurses would say to us, irritated by our complaints. "Can't you understand that?"

Oh forgive us, that makes it all so much better, I would think. A disoriented man watching me shower was certainly forgivable. The fact that they didn't recognize our discomfort with this added loss of privacy made me feel all the more insignificant. Should I have lost all my modesty along with my mind?

Brent and I, both recently having reached A.L. 4 (able to come and go with another "4" or "5," or a friend, staff or family member), decided to take a short walk into Westwood. I wanted to buy some surprises for the girls and Brent, who had been an architectural student, wanted to buy some books. As we were walking, he began to point out things. Things that I couldn't see.

"Look at that fire!" he said, excited. "It will be a long time before they can put that one out. Shit, did you see that accident? That car was totaled!"

My mind flashed back on the MMPI, that weird questionnaire. The question, "I see things or animals or people around me that others do not see."

"Brent, listen, I need to head back. I forgot my money. Can you believe it?"

"No!" he said harshly. "You will not."

"Brent, listen …"

"No, *you* listen. The time has come, the time is right!"

For you to give me a terrible fright, I finished to myself, thinking of Dr. Seuss.

"I am going to include you in a tremendous secret, Kathleen," he whispered.

"O.K., let's start walking back as we talk," I spouted nervously.

"No!" he screamed, grabbing my arm. "Listen to me. I am Satan. You won't believe me now, but you will in time. I'll prove it to you. And I have chosen you as my lady of darkness. We will rule the universe together. We will ..."

What was I doing in Westwood with this person, I wondered. And why was he allowed out of the psychiatric ward? And why had he always seemed relatively normal? And, most important, *why me*?

Brent began to chant—I had no idea what he was saying. He began to rock back and forth in time with his chanting. I began to walk slowly toward the hospital. He stepped in beside me. Terrified, I walked quickly, never craving the surroundings of the locked ward more.

As we were buzzed through the locked door, Brent was quiet. I was shaking all over, and immediately sought out Brent's nurse.

"I just came back from a walk with Brent. He's sick. He's off the deep end. He terrified me. How could you allow him off the ward? How could you do that?"

"Oh, Kathleen, calm down," she said laughing. "If you had any idea of the large number of mentally ill people wandering the streets, you wouldn't be so upset about Brent."

"Well that makes me feel better!" I said, shocked that she was taking this so lightly.

"Brent is harmless, Kathleen," she said placing her hand on my shoulder and becoming serious. "He wouldn't hurt a fly."

As the safety of the ward set in, I felt on the verge of tears. "What's wrong with him?" I asked.

"I can't discuss other patients' cases with you, Kathleen. You know that."

"Will he get better?" I asked, just starting to integrate the evening's events with my affection for Brent.

"Probably not," she said softly. "He's as sick as he is dear."

I was sitting in the day room one afternoon pretending to read a magazine. The ward was nearly empty, with most patients gone to OT—occupational therapy. OT reminded me of the Girl Scouts. We made key chains and pottery and Christmas stockings.

I was staying on the ward this day thinking back on my last experience at OT. A teenage boy from another part of the hospital had been there. He had no hair, was quite thin and extremely pale. He was working on an enormous papier mâché cookie. He was nearly done and very proud. I was deeply touched by his apparent pleasure.

One of the nurses walked by, looked at the cookie and laughed. "It looks pretty real," she said, "but what good is it? It's not like you can use it."

"What good are paintings?" he asked softly. "We just enjoy them. And I had the added pleasure of making this." She walked away and he said, mostly to himself, "And anyway, I'm going to die soon. What 'useful' thing should I have made?"

A tall man in a white jacket came on to the ward. I heard him inquire about Wendy Armstrong. Rumor had it Wendy was from one of the wealthiest families in the United States, suffering from a mental illness no one could classify.

Wendy was brought out to the hallway and Dr. Bell asked her how she was.

"Fine," Wendy answered, "and you?"

Wendy reminded me of a Southern belle on the inside and Boy George on the outside.

"Ah, fine, fine," he said smiling. His manner interested me, and I found his presence extremely comforting. "Should we sit down for a few minutes?" he asked, motioning to the day room, where I already was.

"Certainly," she said graciously.

"So I understand that your family arrived and you had the opportunity to visit with them?" Dr. Bell asked smiling.

"Yes," she said smiling too.

This could take a while, I thought. Some patients cut straight to the core, analyzing themselves and their care for any professional available. But not Wendy.

"And how was the visit?" Dr. Bell asked seeming genuinely interested.

"Fine," Wendy answered.

"Well, what did you talk about?" Dr. Bell asked.

I'd heard comments among the staff about Dr. Bell, the big cheese. "He hardly *ever* comes to this ward." "Try never."

Certainly he had better things to do, I thought. Why couldn't Wendy just answer him?

"Oh the usual," Wendy said, disinterested. She sighed and waved her hand.

"And what was that?" he prodded.

"Oh you know, my mother asked how I was, how's the weather, are there any clipper ships in the area."

"Clipper ships?" Dr. Bell repeated, raising his eyebrows.

"Yes," Wendy said, "clipper ships."

"Ah well," Dr. Bell said warmly, slapping his knee, "that's it then, isn't it?" And he left the ward.

Somewhere in the treatment process years earlier, I'd developed a coping mechanism of always having a current joke or amusing anecdote to distract myself when I felt like crying or screaming or putting my head through a window. Wendy's routine answer, "oh the usual, how's the weather, are there any clipper ships in the area" amused me for weeks to come.

Wendy may not have been able to cut to the chase but Dr. Bell certainly seemed to know when he was beat. "Ah well, that's it then." A knee slap and he was gone.

Turning Point

"Oh yeah, life goes on, long after the thrill of living is gone."

—John Cougar Mellencamp

I remember it slowly dawning on me that because of these experiences in the psych ward I would never be the same. I would never feel carefree or light or laugh freely. There would always be dark undertones. I would not forget all these people and all this pain.

It became clearer and clearer to me that "life is not fair," as I said emotionally, full of self pity, one day to Dr. Jones.

Losing his composure, which I'd never seen him do, he said angrily, "Oh for God's sake Kathleen. Of course it's not! Little kids get cancer and die!"

Slap! I felt foolish. I'd actually been operating on the "Life is fair/ You get what you deserve" theory most of my life. If I was good, good things would come to me. What goes around, comes around. And if it didn't come around in this life then I was surely building credits in heaven.

Accepting that life is not fair was something I needed to do, intellectually and emotionally. I'd been trying to figure out what I'd done to deserve this.

Maybe, I thought, that was less important than what I could do about it.

Dr. Jones now informed me that it had been suggested that I start on an anti-depressant medication. I didn't like taking medication, and the thought of "mind" medication bothered me.

"No amount of medication can stop me from being depressed as long as I'm in pain," I complained.

He could understand my hesitation, Dr. Jones said, but this really was the thing to do.

"Are you sure?" I asked.

"No," he said, "I'm not."

"But it's worth a try?" I asked trying to understand. "Is this your idea?"

"Kathleen, I don't see it as an experiment. And I can't say that it's my idea. I am a resident here. My supervisors, for whom I have the utmost respect, have advised me that this would be an intelligent course of action for a complicated problem. You have a real, serious clinical depression and we need to address it."

"O.K.," I said feeling tense and tired. Once again, I hated the focus on my mental state.

It took many weeks to stabilize me on an anti-depressant. I had various problems with them and figuring out the appropriate type and dosage seemed a kind of hit and miss proposition. The anti-depressants came with all kinds of side effects. I suffered from low blood pressure, dizziness, headaches, constipation, weight gain, and a general fuzzy feeling that I couldn't describe and I couldn't stand. If I thought I'd had no energy previously, was I in for a surprise. I felt heavy, stationary and more confused than ever.

During the afternoons Amanda and Acasia were to visit me, I would sit in the day room trying to "psych" myself up for their visit. Visits with anyone were difficult, visits with the girls being most difficult, because they were the most important. They had so many questions, but they never asked them, having been prompted by Andrew and my mother "not to upset Mommy. Mommy's sick. She can't deal with anything right now." And so there they were, with their childhood imaginations creating far worse scenarios than even existed. Only three and five years old, they had no one talking to them, no adults to make sense of it all. Andrew and my mom were broken, exhausted and confused themselves. They had no idea what to say to them.

The girls needed me more than ever. I was disgusted with myself. I knew I needed to get it together, and I couldn't.

And so my self hate continued to grow. The anger, exhaustion and self hate paralyzed me further.

"How can you wish yourself dead when you love the girls so much?" Andrew asked.

I didn't know. Why did everything have to be black or white, I wondered. How can the area where you had the injection be both numb, and hurt? How can you be in so much pain, and so cautious about possibly addictive pain killers? How can you feel so "heavy" and so "empty?" How can you love your daughters so, and wish yourself dead?

I wanted to say, "I'm the last person to look to for any insight. I'm locked up. Remember?"

Life was so dark. I felt entirely removed, a burden to myself and to others. And I was certain that everyone would be better off without me.

I remember that life struck me as a series of exhausting tasks. I needed to rest after each one. Showering, eating, brushing my teeth, walking, making my bed. The bigger tasks; therapy sessions, physical exams, visits, phone calls or talking with anyone, drained me for hours. And yet you don't cry? the staff would ask. That struck me as an alien thought. What would crying help? It wouldn't change anything. Besides being useless, crying was a personal activity I had given up in the past two years of pain.

Could it be that you feel there are so many tears inside that if you start crying, you imagine it will be like a damn bursting and you may not be able to stop? Dr. Jones asked softly.

I didn't answer.

We were to take turns planning weekend activities. Being both depressed and in pain I felt incapable of committing to something a half hour down the road, let alone for the week-end. My mood seesawed continually based on a change of medication, an unexpected visitor, or a change in my activity level. And sometimes for no apparent reason. Why couldn't they just leave me alone, I wondered. Why did they schedule endless classes such as recreational therapy, occupational therapy, group therapy, assertiveness training classes, singular therapy.

Weekend planning was required as one measure of a patient's progress, I was told by one of the nurses. And so I along with my assigned partner, a U.C.L.A. student in his early twenties "in" for what I assumed was drug addiction, followed through. "Party in your PJ's" was the banner we made in occupational therapy. At our weekly cooking class we made Rice Krispies treats, brownies and chocolate chip cookies. Aren't we progressing, I thought, and I hoped the nursing staff was taking note.

We arrived in the cafeteria Friday night in our PJ's and began a talent show with dances, piano playing, animal imitations and a variety of other talents. For a couple of hours we ate and laughed and it all seemed so "normal." But much too soon the laughter died, and the usual chill set in. In the morning there was no mention of the party.

My mother brought Acasia and Amanda to visit me several times a week. They were not always allowed in, depending on the "conditions of the ward" at the time. The staff had to weigh the effect of the psychiatric ward on small children against the mutual need for us to see each other.

I wrote the girls letters daily, simple factual accounts of the day, expressing my love for them and how much I missed them. I called them several times a week and squirreled away surprises for them any opportunity I had. These simple things drained me. Guilt overwhelmed me. But my depression numbed me.

Mid-October, six weeks after admission: I was sitting in the day room waiting for the girls to visit. I could hardly stay awake. Brent came in. He rarely spoke to anyone, and he never looked like he had much going on in the way of thinking. He seemed dazed, empty. We'd begun our friendship playing ping pong. Neither one of us had any real desire to play ping pong but it was suggested to us that "being sociable" on the ward was helpful to attain more freedom. Freedom as the means for getting off the ward didn't excite me but freedom represented privacy. Being left alone, I thought. That interested me.

We began with ping pong, moved on to backgammon and then minimal talking on the evening ward walks. We both had difficulty finding the energy or words to express ourselves. The anti-depressants still made me fuzzy.

"You'll adjust to them," Dr. Jones promised. "The fuzzy feeling will go away."

It seemed that something wasn't connecting and the simplest thoughts stayed buried. I was fully conscious of them but unable to communicate them. It was a bizarre feeling and one I remember vividly.

At times, the staff or my mother or Andrew would talk about me as if I weren't there.

My friend Carla had visited earlier that day. She'd brought me the latest issue of Vogue magazine. "The new fall issue, Kath. Full of fashion."

Fashion? I repeated to myself. I'd never cared much about "fashion" and I was now locked in a psych ward, caring about very little. Fashion?

Brent pulled a chair up next to mine. "How you doing?" he asked.

People asked me this all day, but when Brent asked he watched my face intently, waiting for a response.

"Amanda and Acasia are coming to visit," I said softly. "I don't want to look like this. Puffy, drugged, a mess."

"Wait here." he said jumping up. He returned quickly, something hidden in his shirt. "Look, smokehouse almonds, a whole can." His face lit up as he revealed them. "Wait here again." he said smiling. "No! Come with me."

We went to the cafeteria and got some coffee (decaf only allowed). The coffee tasted terrible but, "You'll get used to it," old patients promised new patients and we all affectionately referred to it as "bug juice." Back, settled in the day room, the two big orange vinyl chairs pushed side by side we sipped on "bug juice," nibbled smokehouse almonds, and looked page by page at Vogue magazine. We commented on what we liked, what we didn't, and what, if we were the editors, we would have done differently.

I hadn't focused on anything in a long time. And now here it was fall fashions we were looking at. I was startled. Where had the time gone? I'd felt frozen in time, in living hell, for so long now. But I'd subconsciously assumed everyone was. It surprised me that other people's lives were moving along while mine was at a standstill. Or worse, unraveling.

Brent smiled at me. "This is fun Kathy."

"Yeah, it's nice Brent, thank you."

After a long silence he said, "It's the little things Kathy. It's coffee and almonds and a magazine. It's the little things," he repeated, his voice trailing off.

I stayed in the day room, waiting for the girls visit, leafing through miscellaneous newspapers and magazines. The Chinese symbol for crisis, I read, means dangerous opportunity.

Dangerous opportunity. The words kept coming back to me all day.

What could the opportunity be here? I wondered. Dr. Jones and I began to discuss this. Dr. Jones was full of analogies. If I didn't respond to one he'd say, "O.K. forget it," apparently feeling no particular loyalty to any of them. "Let me try again," he'd say. His manner was easy and relaxed. I remember writing somewhere at that time that five minutes with Dr. Jones was "better than a xanax, and there are no side effects."

"Well," Dr. Jones began, "suppose you have a house and it's a fine house, but there's this ugly tree growing right up through the center of it. And you don't have the option of moving or getting rid of the tree. What do you do?"

"Well," I said, "you'd make the rest of the house as beautiful as possible, so that the tree is not the focus."

He smiled and leaned back in his chair.

During my next session with Dr. Jones, I told him that I realized that now the real work was to begin. I knew I had to clean up those areas of my life that I had some control over. I was spending my days looking back at what I could have done to prevent this, or what I might have done to deserve it, rather than at the present and what I could do about it.

"I'm happy to hear you say that, Kathleen. It makes me think of the prayer that goes something like, 'God grant me the serenity to accept the things I cannot change, the courage to change the things I should, and the wisdom to know the difference'," Dr. Jones said.

No more looking back, we agreed. The real issue is what could I now do with my life.

A hell of a lot more than I'd been doing, I realized.

"Very angry with M.D.'s — [Kathleen] will not enter into contract with this M.D. or allow family to be contacted ... Paranoia and anger make therapeutic relationship impossible."

— Hospital records, Dr. Paul Marks

Dr. Jones asked if I was willing to be part of a case conference. I would be interviewed by a psychiatrist at the hospital and other residents, social workers, and nurses would be present.

"Would it help you?" I asked.

"What does that have to do with anything Kathleen?"

"Would it help me?" I responded.

He paused, answering slowly. "Well, I think it might in the sense that we'd have other input as to what might be going on with you Kathleen."

"I'll do it," I said feeling uneasy.

I had become, over the last two years, a guarded patient at best. An angry, suspicious, sarcastic patient at worst. "Paranoid." Being asked the same questions I had already so frequently answered did not excite me. Being asked questions I possessed no answers for tired me. Being made a spectacle bothered me more.

Dr. Keller, the interviewer, impressed me. He asked insightful, sensitive questions. He wanted a glimpse of my childhood, he said. He asked whether either of my parents had been ill while I was growing up. I told him that my father had bleeding ulcers when I was growing up.

"How was that for you?" he asked.

"Unpleasant."

"In what way, Kathleen? Can you tell us a little more about it?"

"I felt that much of our family life focused on his ulcers. We ate what was best for my father, and when it was best for him. We all tiptoed around much of the time afraid to upset him." I continued, telling Dr. Keller that I didn't want to interfere with my daughters' lives in this way. That I didn't want our family life restructured because of my physical problems or limitations.

"And so you are bending over backwards to do the opposite," he said understandingly. "But the fact is that you do have a problem, and you can't sweep it under the rug, or ignore it, or deny it. It would, in fact, be best to accept and deal with it." He questioned my feelings, my general anger, towards the whole medical profession, and then asked about my relationship with Dr. Jones.

Dr. Jones, I said, really did not seem like one of "them" to me. This had never struck me as unusual or significant really, but Dr. Keller seemed quite interested by it.

Sitting in my room, after the case conference I too became interested. Why had our relationship always been an easy one for me? Why was I so ready to see us as a "team?" I remembered my initial impression of him, professional and appropriate. Now another word came to mind. A man. Dr. Jones is a man, I thought with a surge of surprise. I have been sitting, spilling my guts, to a *man*. A young, attractive man to boot. How could I have been too numb to see this?

Maybe the numbing anesthetic of depression began its slow decline that day.

Alternative Medicines

At last it was decided that I was ready to have my first appointment at the pain clinic. The first appointment, that is, since that memorable day weeks earlier, when I'd been told in a most unique manner that I needed to be hospitalized. And so now an escort was sent for me and together we left the ward.

"So, what are you in there for?" asked the young male escort, smiling and motioning back to the ward. I was not much in the mood for conversation and I stared straight ahead, remaining silent. After a short time I made a deliberate effort to smile at him, with the intention of not being entirely rude. Had I wanted to answer him I doubt that I would have known what to say.

"Maybe we could have lunch some day," he said lightheartedly.

"Maybe," I said softly, distracted. The pain clinic was down two levels and clear to the other end of the hospital, a considerable walk. My anxiety began to build. I was embarrassed at returning to a place I'd last been escorted out of by two guards, on my way to being committed.

After a couple of minutes the escort obviously sensed something because he turned to me and gently asked, "Hey, are you all right?"

No, I'm half left, I thought. But I only said, "Yes, I'm fine."

The pain clinic was on the basement level of the hospital. It had no windows and was both poorly furnished and consistently crowded. Immediately upon my arrival on this visit and many of my future visits, I would locate a magazine, any magazine, and sit down. A magazine was fairly effective insurance for being left alone. Then my mind would be off and running. I would think about how poorly organized the pain clinic was, how displeasing the place was aesthetically. And how angry I was to be there as a result of someone else's negligence.

I would be kept waiting without fail and my anger would build, as would my conviction that the medical profession was a group of sadistic incompetents. But for the time being I still believed that they were in control and knew what they were doing, and that I was just a patient.

So when someone called my name, quietly and smiling all the while, I walked to the appropriate room and did whatever was asked of me.

The pain clinic treatments began as they said they would, with the least invasive first. The treatments seemed to increase the cramping and burning. And I came away from them feeling worse.

I had mixed feelings regarding the pain clinic altogether. I was both relieved and grateful to find medical practitioners who believed they could work with me, and not to be met with resignation. And yet in many ways the pain clinic just wasn't structured for people in chronic pain.

We were left waiting, appointments were canceled after we'd already arrived for them, and since this was a teaching facility we were talked about at length even while on the examining table, and examined frequently both in front of medical students and by them.

"They have to learn somewhere," the nurses said haughtily. How about on you? I wanted to say. Yeah, that's it. Let them learn on you.

I told them that my pain level was increasing.

"What do you mean? Don't you really mean that your ability to deal with it is lessening?"

"No, I mean the pain is increasing."

"The pain is not increasing, Kathleen, your tolerance of it is decreasing. You will find that one thing we will be able to help you with here, even if we are unable to affect your pain level, is the 'bothersomeness' of your pain. While the pain may remain the same, you will learn how to reduce the bothersomeness."

I thought they were nuts.

Let's try a tens unit, was the first suggestion. "Tens" stands for "transcutaneous electrical neural stimulation." The unit looked a little like a transistor radio and sent small electrical pulses to targeted areas as a distraction from the pain and also hopefully as a stimulus for the production of endorphins. The pain increased.

"What do you mean the pain increases?" the physical therapist asked, annoyed.

"The area where I had the injection begins to cramp more," I said.

"Oh Kathleen, how can it hurt more? It doesn't hurt more. What are we going to do with you? What is it you want us to do with you?"

Slitting my throat might be nice.

Next was massage therapy and acupressure. Again the pain increased.

How about acupuncture? they asked. Clearly they're not thinking straight I thought. This all *began* with a needle.

With tremendous anxiety I agreed to acupuncture treatments, only to back out, petrified, on my first appointment.

"Oh Kathleen, be reasonable. Acupuncture is not an injection, for goodness sake."

"Good point," I said frustrated. "What is acupuncture? How does it work? Why does it work? In fact, does it work? Will we soon have some crystals in here, and maybe do some chanting?"

"No one knows how acupuncture works Kathleen, or if it will work. But you're the one with the pain."

Yes, I was the one with the pain.

"I'll try it." I said wearily.

But I couldn't go through with it. I saw the acupuncturist walk in with a handful of needles and I asked to be taken back to the ward. "I'm a loser," I told Dr. Jones that night during our session. "Instead of sitting here telling you about my acupuncture appointment I am telling you what a chicken I was. I'm paranoid about needles," I continued, "I just can't do it."

"You are not 'paranoid' about needles Kathleen. And you can do it. You were nervous. Anyone would be. It was new. New things can be scary."

Yeah, that's it. I was nervous. Not paranoid. Not a loser. Nervous. Dr. Jones consistently re-labeled my feelings in a more positive light. The negative silent messages I'd been giving myself were quite powerful. I needed to find new silent messages that would generate health rather than sickness.

Within days I was undergoing acupuncture treatments. I'd been promised I "would never know" the needles were there. I knew. They didn't hurt, but were uncomfortable and I couldn't relax. The physical therapist used a small hammer-like device to gently tap the needles through my skin. The idea, let alone the action, upset me. In addition I noticed no positive effect from the treatments.

"How about massage therapy? And diaphragmatic breathing?" the physical therapist asked me.

"Diaphragmatic breathing?" I asked.

"Yes, Kathleen. Put your hand on your abdomen and take a deep breath in. Does your abdomen go in or out?"

"In," I answered.

"Exactly. Now if you went home and put your hand on either of your children's abdomens, I imagine the answer would be out. We all begin life breathing properly. Somewhere along the line, due to tension or whatever, we do the opposite."

"So what?"

"So you will find diaphragmatic breathing is very relaxing, and helpful to someone suffering from chronic pain."

Diaphragmatic breathing, I repeated to myself. Hmm, I thought, they tell me here at the pain management center that they understand my pain, and that they think they can help. They tell me that the pain that I am experiencing is comparable to that of someone with terminal cancer. And now they suggest massage therapy and breathing lessons?

"How about hypnosis Kathleen? Are you willing?"

Not again! Here I was at U.C.L.A., a well respected hospital and university, and they wanted to treat physical pain with hokey pokey? Acupuncture was pushing it, but hypnosis? I was nervous. But if hokey pokey was my only option I wasn't about to dismiss it. Dr. Jones urged me to try it. We were rapidly building the kind of relationship in which had he urged me to walk on water, I would have tried.

Hypnosis was amazing, like magic really. Somehow I'd thought that I would have to "believe" for it to work. I'd thought that I would basically be unconscious and unaware of what went on. Not so. I remembered what the hypnotist said, my response, and my feelings, vividly. She brought me back to my childhood in New Hampshire. I was in a field of flowers with my cousins, and our family dog. It was believable and extraordinarily relaxing.

I was ecstatic. I could hardly contain myself when I next saw Dr. Jones. "It worked!" I nearly shrieked. "I relaxed and when we were done I felt like I'd slept for hours. I'm happy and hopeful," I said smiling. "I haven't felt relaxed or rested for a long time, and I'd forgotten how magical some things are."

"Well, good," Dr. Jones said smiling. "I was told things went well Kathleen. I'm pleased. Everyone is. I guess I've never seen you this excited."

"You haven't," I said dryly. "But then I'm in a psych ward. There aren't that many opportunities."

"O.K., O.K.," he said smiling, "Would you like Patricia to teach you self hypnosis? To aid in stress reduction?"

"I don't think I would know how," I said feeling doubtful.

"You're a perfect candidate for it Kathleen," he assured me.

"O.K., let's try," I said with a surge of excitement.

Patricia arrived at our next session with a tape recorder. I stiffened. "I thought we could make a tape for you to practice with, Kathleen. You won't be on the tape, only me," she added, sensing my tension.

The session was brief and productive.

"You have homework," she said smiling when we were done. "I want you to practice by listening to this tape a couple of times a day," she said. "If it doesn't work right away, don't worry. It *will* work. Dr. Jones will let you know when we've arranged your next appointment."

I played the tape in bed at night with headphones and within a few days I was noticing a sense of relaxation from it. But I was embarrassed to be learning self hypnosis. It all seemed so "California." It reminded me of Woody Allen ordering a bowl of brewers yeast, or alfalfa sprouts, or whatever, in Annie Hall. Now I was "seeing" someone for therapy "sessions." I'd tried acupuncture. And now a hypnotist.

During our next session Patricia said, "O.K., we've been quite successful, and we've moved quickly, so I thought today we would try something new. Would that be all right with you Kathleen?"

"Sure," I said agreeable immediately. This hypnosis stuff is remarkable, I thought.

She said we would try "guided imagery," which sounded to me as if we would be taking an armchair vacation together. She put me "under" and away we went. She suggested that I see myself on a beach. "Do you see it?" she asked. "Do you smell the sea air and hear the waves hitting the shore? Do you feel the warmth of the sand? O.K., good."

"Now," she said, "I want you to begin digging in the sand." I did this. I said nothing. "Kathleen, are you digging?"

"Yes," I answered distracted, beginning to tense. "Good, now keep digging. And tell me what you discover there. Something is buried there, waiting for you. Just waiting for you to find it."

"I don't want to dig anymore," I said. "I think it's time to stop."

"No, Kathleen. I want you to tell me what you uncover as you continue to dig."

"I can't." I felt a knot in my stomach and I was scared.

"You need to do this, Kathleen," Patricia said. "It's important."

"It's not a good idea. I don't want to do this. I need to stop."

"Kathleen, we need to do this."

Now I could see, quite clearly, why I'd felt anxious and wanted to stop. Here in this pit I was digging in the sand, was blood. A huge pool of blood. What should I do? I wondered. As horrible as it all was I wanted to understand what was going on. And as I continued digging there were fragments. Of what? "I need to stop now." I could barely get the words out.

"No Kathleen," Patricia said, gently prodding me. "We need to see what is there waiting for you. What is it Kathleen?"

An arm, a leg, a foot. I thought I was going to vomit. Oh my God! What have I discovered? Now there was blood on me. I was covered with it. The hole was increasing in size rapidly, all by itself, and filling with blood. Now the waves were washing in. More blood. My whole body was covered and it wouldn't wipe off. The hole was probably ten times its original size now and rapidly increasing. The blood was a vibrant red, and there must have been hundreds of body parts floating on top. My whole body began to shake and I began to moan. I shot straight up in bed. "I can't do this anymore," I screamed. And now here was Patricia looking at me wide eyed, critical, interested. Every inch of me said get it together Kathy, get a hold of yourself. "I don't like hypnosis. It's not working for me," I spat out.

"Kathleen, what's wrong? " Patricia asked, taken aback. She moved towards me and I pulled away, pulling the covers of the bed up around my neck. "Talk to me. We can work through this together. But you need to let me in," she continued.

I let you in, I thought, and look what you have done to me, look where you have taken me. "I don't want to talk," I said, putting tremendous effort into not getting "hysterical." Locked up in a psych ward, I was sensitive to the fact that most of what I said and did was being monitored, judged. I was afraid. Afraid of the very system that was, it appeared, my only avenue for hope. I didn't want to seem anything worse than I already had been labeled. I stood on my head to appear in control. I wanted to say, how could you do this to me? How could you lead me to believe that I was going to achieve relaxation and a better knowledge of my inner whatever, and take me to a bloody pit and have me dig in it, surrounding myself with severed limbs and cover myself in blood?

"Kathleen," she said with a forced calm, "you need to let me take you out of the trance. You can't just stop like this. You'll develop a headache, you'll feel anxious..."

Tell me about it, I was thinking. My head felt split in two, on fire. I thought I may vomit, and I felt the blood all over me and wanted to shower desperately. "O.K.," I said and laid back down. I couldn't let go though. I couldn't concentrate and I didn't trust her.

"Kathleen, we need to discuss what upset you," Patricia said when it became obvious that I wasn't going to go back under. "What scared you?"

"I don't want to discuss it. I don't want to talk. I want to stop now. I want to be alone. I'm fine." She continued questioning me, but I was no help. I didn't want to discuss what I'd uncovered, what "scared" me, especially not with the very person that set me up for it.

Patricia left, obviously unhappy with my lack of cooperation. A couple of nurses came in "just to see how you're doing," having been alerted by Patricia that I wasn't doing well. I didn't want to talk. I wanted to shower, but I was drained and shaky and nauseous. And so I lay there in the fetal position, in a pool of blood, shivering, wanting to die.

Dr. Jones came almost running into my room. "Kathleen," he said, breathless, looking shaken and concerned, "I just heard. Are you all right? How do you feel? Can you walk to my office? Will you talk to me?"

The heaviness and feeling of doom began to lift. I wanted to cry. I remembered one day when I was in first grade, I'd gone to the nurse's office at school, not feeling well. The nurse had tucked me into a cot and left to call my mother. I laid there hearing doors open and close and the phone ring, and I was quiet. I was left there waiting for what seemed like forever. Maybe she'd forgotten me. Maybe she'd forgotten to call my mother. What if I throw up here and the school nurse gets mad at me? What if they can't reach my mother? And all of a sudden my mother appeared, capable and pretty and concerned, and I filled with relief. What took you so long? I whispered and she hugged me tight.

Shaky, I walked to his office. Slowly I discussed with Dr. Jones what I'd uncovered in the sand. I felt embarrassed that my mind had created such a sick place. "I don't like hypnosis," I told him. "I don't want to do it anymore."

"I imagine you don't," he said. "And you don't have to." That was all he said. He didn't ask me what I thought the blood, or bodily parts meant. He didn't ask me why I wasn't willing to discuss this with Patricia. He didn't tell me that it would be good for me to continue my hypnosis sessions with Patricia. Or that we would certainly have to get to the bottom of what all this meant. "She had no right to pursue 'guided imagery' with you Kathleen. She was supposed to teach you relaxation techniques. Not delve, barely knowing you, into who knows what. I'm sorry it happened, Kathleen."

A few days later Dr. Jones and I had another conversation about the guided imagery episode. I was calmer now. In fact I was calmer that first night, just having seen Dr. Jones. He now said that since hypnosis had originally proven to be so successful at reducing my stress level, I had the option of continuing with Patricia, on the original plan. Self hypnosis. That she had been instructed not to veer off of her original set of instructions. That there was absolutely no pressure for me to do this, but that since I'd had a positive reaction to it initially it might be a good idea. I agreed. I surprised myself in doing this. The last episode with the pool of body parts and blood that wouldn't wash off was still vivid in my mind.

Patricia and I met, or should I say she came to my hospital room, once again. I laid down and she sat in a chair next to my bed. The door of the room was closed with a "DO NOT DISTURB!" sign posted. She put me "under" and I began to relax. Suddenly in burst a nurse screaming about something.

"Can't you see the 'Do Not Disturb' sign on the door?" Patricia shouted. I sat up quickly, my head throbbing. The nurse, embarrassed blurted out an apology and closed the door quickly. "It's O.K., Kathleen," Patricia said. "Lay back, and we'll continue."

But I couldn't continue. Now or ever, I told Patricia.

"Don't you want to get better?" Patricia asked.

"I just can't do this," I said haltingly.

She left. I didn't see Patricia again but I did continue to use the self hypnosis tape in bed at night and it proved to be immensely helpful in relaxing me just enough to fall asleep.

November 8, 1984: I decided I had to go home. In a frenzy I informed Dr. Jones of this, and began to pack. Dr. Jones tried to reason with me. No way. I wanted to go home.

"I've been here over two months and look at the shape I'm in." I spat at him. "I'm a drugged zombie, and you know what's funny? " I continued. "I'm paying a fortune to have this done to me. I hate it here and I want to go home."

Dr. Jones looked uncomfortable. "I know this isn't an easy place to be Kathleen, but you need to be here. I certainly can't release you at this point."

"Release me? If you don't want to sign the release papers, that's fine. I've been here long enough to know I can sign out A.M.A. (against medical advice)."

All compassion drained from Dr. Jones' face — he had for the first time since I'd met him, a strictly business expression. Dr. Jones informed me that I couldn't go home and if I attempted to leave he would have to put a "hold" on me. That's something, he said, he didn't want to do. A "hold" meant I couldn't go home or anywhere else for that matter. And that my activity level would be reduced to a 1, confined to the ward for 72 hours for observation purposes. The idea of being under heavier observation made my skin crawl.

I was sick of having everything I brought into the ward searched, and having a flashlight shined in my face at night to chart whether or not I was sleeping, and having a nurse sit staring while I ate to chart my eating habits. I was sick of having blood drawn for God knows what purpose, and sick of group therapy, "community" meetings and week-end planning.

"You're a bunch of nuts yourselves," I told Dr. Jones. "Just the fact that you would do this to depressed people. Are you trying to push us over the edge? Have you ever tasted the crap they expect us to eat? And if we don't we're suspected, as in my case, of possible anorexia, and we're watched even more closely. I want to be with Amanda and Acasia. I want out. Can't you see that?"

"I can see that you are very upset Kathleen." Dr. Jones said.

Well now, that's observant, I mused.

"I want what's best for you, Kathleen," Dr. Jones continued. "And right now I think you need to be somewhere safe. We can talk tomorrow if you are calm but in the meantime you will not be permitted to leave the ward. Good night," he said looking exhausted and unhappy.

I felt a stab of guilt and was unhappy to have rocked our previously smooth doctor-patient relationship. But then I looked around at the ward and I hated him, the hospital, life, and mostly myself. Well, there you go I thought, this place is not a hotel you check in and out of but more like a roach motel — "You check in but you can't check out."

By late that evening I knew that Dr. Jones did want what was best for me. I was embarrassed.

"Don't mention it," he said the next morning, waving his hand, dismissing it. "We all have our days," he said smiling. "Now let's talk about what we need to work on so you *can* go home. And be ready for it."

I appreciated that he said "we" all have our days, not "you." It had been my observation while hospitalized that the majority of the staff felt a strong need to separate themselves from their patients, physically, emotionally and therapeutically.

Family

About two weeks later, Dr. Jones decided not only that I could but that I should go home.

"I couldn't agree more," I said beaming.

"I'm sorry we couldn't reduce the pain Kathleen, but your depression has begun to clear up, which was our immediate concern. My understanding through talking to the pain management center is that you will continue on an out patient basis with them, and of course we've agreed you will continue seeing me twice a week."

I was disappointed that I'd entered the hospital for what I'd expected to be a week, spent nearly three months instead, and was experiencing the same level of pain I had been when I was admitted. But I had to admit, my mood had slowly begun to improve. I was far from feeling happy, but now I had occasional glimpses of gray where before there had only been black.

"I'm grateful you're willing to see me on an outpatient basis, Dr. Jones. I have a hard time thinking that us sitting here talking twice a week will do much for me, though. I'd rather I had no pain."

"Well, I would too Kathleen. There's no question about that. In the absence of that option however, I think therapy will prove to be quite useful for you. And I'm looking forward to working with you."

And so a couple of days before Thanksgiving and three months after I admitted myself to the psych ward, I returned home.

The separation from Andrew hadn't given us a breather, a chance to miss each other as I'd hoped. Instead our problems multiplied. While hospitalized, the direction I was taking changed. Previous to it, I wanted what Andrew wanted — to be the way I used to be. Andrew and I had together resented members of the medical profession suggesting I learn to live with the pain. We'd both agreed that if we tried hard enough and long enough we could fix me and return to life as we knew it.

Mid-way through my hospitalization, I began to understand that it was unlikely they could fix me, and unlikely we would ever regain the life we'd known. And by my discharge date I knew that even if a miracle took place, and the pain vanished, my experiences had permanently changed me. It became clear to me that I needed to get to know the new me, despite my limitations, my moods, my seriousness.

"Well, I don't like you this way!" Andrew said, slapping his hand down on the table in front of him, my second day home.

"Neither do I, *yet*," I said. "But that's the point. We need to work on it."

"What happened to you when you were in there, Kathy? I thought we agreed that the whole point of you going in there in the first place was to get better."

"Actually, the real reason I went in there, Andrew, was so that I wouldn't kill myself. Remember?"

"Yeah, and to straighten yourself out. But then you got all chummy with everybody and forgot why you were there. When I brought you there the first day, you hated it. But then you began greeting everybody like they were your best friends, like *they* understood. You got pretty comfortable there, Kathy, didn't you?"

"I certainly wasn't comfortable Andrew. And they weren't my best friends. But to a certain extent, they did understand what I was going through, better than you could. Just like *their* husbands or wives or whatever would understand what it was like for *you* having your wife locked up, better than I could."

"Yeah, and now you're talking like one of those doctors you used to hate. Now you're saying you have to 'accept your limitations.' Before you went into the hospital, we had enough problems. But at least we were headed in the same direction. We wanted the same thing. Now you want me to accept you sick like this, forever. Well I don't want to. I want a *wife*!"

"You have a wife, Andrew," I said sadly. "Just not a desirable one."

No longer headed in the same direction, we now argued daily.

Andrew felt he was supportive of me because he was there with me — I felt there was more to support than bodily presence. I felt inadequate and angry. Financial pressures were mounting, and so accordingly were the amount of hours Andrew worked at construction weekly. I felt guilty beyond compare.

Andrew refused counseling. I felt counseling was our only chance. "What the hell do we need a counselor for Kathy?" he'd say looking old and tired. "Can they change anything? Can they pay our bills ? Or just add to them? We can talk between ourselves."

"But we don't talk, Andrew. We argue."

"Anybody would fight with you, Kathy. You feel miserable all of the time. Just looking at you makes me feel miserable. And now you want me to see a therapist? Well, I don't believe in therapists, and even if I did I don't have the time. I'm working around the clock to pay your bills and now you want me to take time off so we can sit and talk to somebody about things we can't change? We do have some control over our finances and I'd rather concentrate on them. Be reasonable, Kathy," he said, his voice cracking. "When the hell would I go?"

And so I said I'd leave.

"Leave?" Andrew shouted. "For Christ's sake Kathy. I don't know whether to laugh or to cry. We have no money, you were just released from a mental ward. You don't even have a job. How the hell do you think you're going to take care of the girls? Do you know how lonely you would be?"

"I'm lonely now," I said gritting my teeth.

"You're what?"

"I'm lonely now. Are you really working all the time you're away Andrew? Or are you trying to get away from me?"

"I'm trying," he said angrily, "to pay your bills. You amaze me Kathy, do you know that? You complain of pain that no one can see, have a nervous breakdown, get us into financial straits, and now accuse me of trying to get away because I'm working all the time? You're *lonely*? "

"Even when you're home, I'm lonely," I said, the words just slipping out, and the cold, awful truth hitting us.

"What the hell is that supposed to mean?" Andrew asked incredulously.

"Andrew, we don't talk. You just keep telling me we'll talk when I'm the way I 'used to be.' I feel lonelier living with you, with absolutely no communication, than I would being physically alone."

"How do you know that?" he said furious.

"I don't. But if you won't go to counseling with me, I guess I'll find out," I said coldly.

"You're just trying to destroy us, aren't you?" he shouted. "I get it! You're not trying to save our marriage, are you? You're on a self destruct mission. What is wrong with you anyway?"

I wished I knew.

My hospital stay had affected the girls dramatically. They were afraid to let me out of their sight. And so they accompanied me everywhere. They watched me brush my teeth, shower, sleep, and most certainly attend doctor appointments — even if it meant waiting outside with my mom, as they did during therapy sessions. I wasn't going to get locked up again. Not if they had anything to do with it.

Acasia and Amanda were always remarkably well behaved. It was rare that I would take them anywhere without someone remarking on this. Now they were too good though and it worried me. I knew they were concerned that I'd get sick again and they'd taken it upon themselves to be sure I didn't. Talking to them did little to relieve this. I told them over and over that nothing they had done had made me sick, and that nothing they did could make me better. That I was the adult, and that I was both responsible for and capable of getting myself together. Slowly, very slowly they began to believe me.

I told them that it was important that they let their bad feelings out. And that not only was it expected that on some level that they would be angry with me for abandoning them, but that it was quite healthy to be.

"In fact," I said, "I'd be surprised if you weren't furious with me for leaving you while I was in the hospital. So furious that you wished harm on me. And then maybe you felt guilty. Well you shouldn't. It's o.k. Nothing will happen to mommy as a result."

"Oh good," Amanda said with an enormous sigh of relief. And then I knew we were getting somewhere, together.

It wasn't working. I've been to the city, I've seen the white elephant, I thought. Why was I still floundering? I knew I had to take responsibility for myself, for my health. "Dangerous opportunity," I kept repeating to myself. What could I try now?

I began to think of Joanne, a nurse, who'd urged me, several times, to see Dr. Steven Rosenblatt, an acupuncturist she'd seen. "You'll love him," she said. "He's warm and kind and gentle. So, when are you going to make an appointment with him? " she asked.

Well, how about when hell freezes over — that seems as good a time as any to pay someone to stick me with needles again. "Do you remember that I already tried acupuncture here at U.C.L.A.? And it was an awful experience, as well as of no help."

Eventually hell froze over. I called Dr. Rosenblatt's office and set an appointment. I guessed that I would benefit more from the hope that stemmed from trying something new than that I would suffer from the fear.

Dr. Rosenblatt talked with me for a long time, examined me, and then talked to me again. "It's pretty straightforward, Kathleen. I wish I'd seen you soon after the injury. Three years later is a long time. "

I was silent.

"But I still think I can help."

"You think it's straightforward and that you can help, Dr. Rosenblatt?" I began to smile.

"You don't think it's strange or unusual or confusing? I mean my leg is numb but it hurts. You don't find this strange? And I have complaints from head to toe, not just where I had the injection."

"I'd say that it's law conforming with the type of injury you have."

Law conforming. I liked that.

He recommended that I read the book, "DLPA To End Chronic Pain and Depression." "Depression goes right along with chronic pain, Kathleen. DLPA, dl phenylalanine, is an amino acid used for the treatment of both. I want you to get some immediately."

I was pleased that he wanted to treat my depression *along* with my pain.

I picked up the amino acid, read the book, and also began drinking aloe vera juice, which was referred to in the book. Aren't you supposed to put that on burns and things? a neighbor suggested. Not drink it!

Well, it's worth a try, I said, shrugging my shoulders. If the extract from the plant helps topically it makes sense that it could help the nerve injury if the juice is taken internally.

"You'll try anything, huh Kath?"

Just about, I thought feeling exhausted.

Acupuncture treatments began. Much to my surprise I couldn't even feel the needles going in. Why had it hurt so much previously, I asked Dr. Rosenblatt, and why had the previous acupuncturist used that little metal hammer to insert the needles?

"There's more than one type of acupuncture treatment Kathleen," is all he said.

I saw improvement quickly — as far as my headaches were concerned. However it only seemed to aggravate the area where I'd had the injection.

"I would expect that Kathleen," Dr. Rosenblatt said reassuringly. "Often it feels worse before it feels better."

It's always darkest before the dawn. What goes up must come down. You can't fix the problems of a year in a day. What goes around comes around. If it's not one thing it's another, I thought wearily.

Dr. Rosenblatt didn't treat a part of me. He treated me, Kathleen, as a whole, taking an interest in my overall health.

I had become accustomed to being embarrassed by my long list of physical complaints and my new history of clinical depression. I wanted to answer doctors questions fully and accurately, but they usually seemed busy, hurried. I didn't know what was an important part of my medical history and what wasn't. The doctors would grow seemingly impatient with my history, and my embarrassment and frustration would build.

Dr. Rosenblatt appeared to have the time and the interest for my complete medical history on my first appointment, and at every appointment thereafter was relaxed and unhurried.

"Is anything on your mind Kathleen? Do you have any questions?" he'd always ask. The girls went with me to see him and he always talked to the three of us gently and kindly, seeming in tune with their painful concern for my health. Chalk one more up for the medical profession, I thought.

I saw Dr. Rosenblatt two or three times a week, continued therapy sessions with Dr. Jones twice a week, and kept up various pain clinic appointments. In addition I felt in a panic to make up for lost time with the girls. They were growing so quickly. I resented the time I'd missed with them, and I wanted to get us back on the right track.

Things continued to deteriorate between Andrew and me however.

He would alternately promise to get therapy or become furious when I would suggest it. Once when he was supposed to meet me at U.C.L.A. for a session with Dr. Jones, he called to say his truck had broken down.

"The truck broke down Andrew? It took you over a year to agree to *one* therapy session and the *truck broke down*?"

"Yes it did Kathy," Andrew said angrily. "I wanted to see Dr. Jones as much as you wanted me to."

"Good, then when can we reschedule for?" I asked.

"Sorry Kath, I can't reschedule right now. And anyway, why should I get counseling for *your* problem?"

"It's *our* problem, Andrew."

"If we could just go back to our old life, Kathy."

"But that's the problem Andrew," I said, my voice raising. "Don't you get it? We can't."

"Not until you grow up, we can't, Kathy," he said, his voice flooding with anger.

"Grow up? Andrew, what the hell is that supposed to mean?"

"Forget I said it," he said sighing.

"If you tell the truth you don't have to remember anything."

—Mark Twain

In August 1985, as part of the discovery for my eventual trial, Andrew's deposition was taken. Before we met with the opposing attorney, Neil met with us. He said he knew we'd been through a lot, and that we shouldn't worry about the deposition. He said that many of the questions would be routine, and that we should answer to the best of our ability, truthfully and in a concise manner.

He asked Andrew if he had any recollection of the emergency room episode. Andrew said he remembered quite well.

"Did you witness the injection?" Neil asked.

"No," Andrew said.

"But did you see the injection site afterwards?"

"Yes, I did."

"Do you clearly recall that site?"

"I do. I remember a little prick of blood."

"Do you remember what happened that night, who you spoke to, what Kathleen said and did?"

"Yes, it's etched in my brain."

"Terrific," Neil said. "This part of your testimony will be significant — the remainder will be much less important. Your memory of that night is a strong factor in this deposition, in the outcome of Kathleen's case actually. Do you understand that, Andrew?"

"I do."

As Andrew and I walked down the corridor to the deposition room, Andrew said to me softly, "If you win this case Kathy, you'll have the money to leave me. If you lose you just might try to work things out."

"What is that supposed to mean?" I asked Andrew confused.

"It means," he said, "that your case is a sure bet. And you stand to win a lot of money..."

"*We* stand to be awarded a lot of money." I interjected.

"Enough money," he repeated as though to himself, "to leave me."

"Were you present for any portion of time," the defense attorney asked Andrew, "during which your wife received treatment in the emergency room at Columbus Memorial Hospital in April of 1982?"

"No," Andrew replied.

"So you did not see any treatment rendered to her; is that correct?"

"Correct."

"Did you talk with any doctor at Columbus Memorial Hospital that evening?"

"I remember the nurse and I think I remember the doctor coming in, but — I don't know."

"Did you talk to your wife about the emergency room treatment the evening it was rendered?"

"Yes."

"What did she tell you?"

"She said she felt like they hit a bone and it hurt her quite a bit."

"Did she tell you anything else?"

"She did, but I can't remember. We talked about it and — It's just so long ago now that I just can't get a clear picture."

That's it? My head started to spin. I felt dizzy. I wanted to scream. Is this where I wake up? I hoped, gasping for air. Everyone was quiet, as I sat there shaking, although the defense counsel had a distinct look of satisfaction on her face.

"Andrew, how could you do that to me?" I asked the minute we were in the car.

"Do what?" he said, his face pale, with a vague trace of a smile. "I didn't *do* anything."

"Andrew, you've ruined everything. First you tell Neil the night of the injection is 'etched in your brain.' Neil tells you that your memory of that night is a strong factor in the outcome of the case. Suddenly the deposition begins and you tell them it's just so long ago 'you can't get a clear picture.'"

"I did it for us Kathy. Can't you understand that? I did it for us."

"Will you see a therapist *now*, Andrew?" I asked.

"Besides the fact that I don't have the time or the money, I think it's a waste of time," he said stone-faced. "Besides," he softened, "I'm scared."

"Scared?" I repeated dumfounded. "Of what?"

"Well, I've been having some crazy thoughts myself," he said slowly. "When you were locked up, it scared me. You made it through and out of that crazy place. I don't think I could do it."

"You don't need to," I said confused. "Nobody's locking you up."

"Well, they might if they knew what I was thinking," he said, his shoulders sagging, voice heavy.

Well, that's comforting, I thought.

"Look, we've both been under stress." I said taking his hand. "All of us have. Together we could try to work it out. Do you realize that we never talk?"

"We have nothing to talk about," he said taking his hand away.

"We can talk about our future," I said.

"Kathy, all the talking in the world won't accomplish what you need to do."

"Which is?"

"Be the person I married —"

"Oh Andrew …"

"It's true Kathy. I hate who you've become. And now all you tell me is *I* need counseling. Why are you so obsessed with counseling, anyway?"

"I don't give a fuck about counseling, Andrew. It's the *reason* we need counseling I'm 'obsessed' with."

"And what's that?"

"Andrew, you say you hate who I've become. You say you hate the loss of my innocence and laughter, and physical and emotional well being. Well, the loss is as much mine as yours. I know how hard this has been, and you have been wonderful. But you continually remind me that you don't like me now. Would you expect a Vietnam Vet to come home and be silly and carefree, the way he used to be?"

"You didn't go to war, Kathy," Andrew said exasperated.

"No but I've been through hell. And if I'm ever going to be o.k., I can't live with a person who doesn't like who I am now. Together, maybe we can learn to like who I've become, and to build a new life together. A *different* life."

"Guess what, Kathy? I don't want a new life. And I sure don't want to get used to you this way. So why don't you just concentrate on yourself instead of playing psychiatrist with me."

I told Andrew I was leaving.

"How can you leave me Kathy, when I love you so much," he said softly, his voice cracking.

I had no answer. Anger and exhaustion overwhelmed me

"What about the girls?" he asked. "How can you do this to them?"

I'd asked myself this a thousand times already. But when I finally stopped and played it through, the mixed message I would be giving the girls by staying seemed far more damaging.

I didn't love Andrew anymore. I didn't think he loved me either. I wished we were still in love.

"You'll love me again Kathy. I know you will. Give it a chance. Give us a chance. It would kill me Kathy — the thought of you out with someone else."

"I have no interest in dating, Andrew. And anyway I don't think guys will be knocking my door down. I'm a mess."

"Well there you go, Kathy. I want you. I want to take care of you. You need me. Think about it. There's no getting around it, you're mentally ill. I mean Kathy… you just spent three months in a psychiatric ward."

"Is that what that was?"

"Why are you so cold now?" Andrew asked angrily.

Years of pain and litigation are funny that way, I thought. They take that tender, caring part of you and turn it to rock.

"Promise me one thing," Andrew continued. "You won't date anyone. I'd kill myself. Are you listening Kathy?"

"You wouldn't kill yourself."

"I would kill you."

"You wouldn't kill yourself," I repeated distracted.

"I said I would kill *you*," he said, a far away look in his eyes.

"You would kill me, Andrew?" I said laughing. "Where were you when I needed you?"

"You're so cold now, and everything is so funny to you Kathy. Well, I'd stop laughing if I was you."

Laughter has always been a coping mechanism for me. I was always embarrassed to laugh at inappropriate times, but I preferred it to crying. "Why do you think that is?" Dr. Jones asked, "that you prefer laughing to crying?"

"Don't most people?" I replied. However, as Andrew began to emotionally slide, along with any small hope I had of ever mending our relationship, the laughter died.

On September 27, 1985, my 29th birthday, I borrowed $3,000 from my sister and rented a tiny, rundown one bedroom apartment.

"You have to do what you have to do Kath," Neil said throwing up his hands when he heard I'd moved out. "But this isn't going to help your case. I told you that. The jurors will feel for you and Andrew together. Having left him you may just come across as a bitch. First the psychiatric hospitalization, and now this. I don't know, Kath," he said, his voice trailing off.

"Why do I have to worry about the jurors?" I asked in disbelief. "Both the hospitalization and the separation are a result of stress stemming from the injection Neil. That's just part and parcel of the law suit, I would think."

The Ladies Room

One of the nurses in the hospital had said one evening, "Kathleen, if you and your daughters were lost in the woods, no food, by yourselves—and you were all hungry, but you only had a tiny bit of food left, what would you do with it?"

"Divide it between my daughters," I answered, wondering why people ask such ridiculous questions.

"Wrong answer," he said matter of factly. "*You* should eat it. Because without you they wouldn't have a prayer. You'd need to conserve your strength so that you could care for them. Protecting yourself would be their protection."

The years of stress since the injection were something Andrew and I couldn't handle together. "Well if you couldn't be there for each other in the tough times, it's good you know now." Or, "If you had that much trouble communicating you couldn't have made it together anyway." Or, "Look, you married too young, eighteen years old. What did you expect?"

Maybe. But Andrew and I had proven ourselves equipped to handle the normal pressures of a young family just starting out. The injection-related stress was too much. Many couples break up as a result of far less stress and others stay together in the midst of more.

"Heroes are those with the courage to leave what they have ...not without fear, but without succumbing to their fear."

—Erich Fromm

I had always thought that fear was a signal like acute pain. Danger, warning, cease activity. I now needed to remind myself continually that this was not the case.

I remember the first day I brought the girls to our new "home." I was nervous. I'd fixed it up with the help of friends and family, but nevertheless it was a rundown one bedroom apartment, not a four bedroom house. And there was very little furniture. Amanda, age six and a half, and Acasia, age four and a half, walked in and looked all around silently. Wide eyed they wandered around looking in every nook and cranny. "It's empty," Amanda said softly. My stomach was churning. "Lots of room to ride our bikes," she said breaking into a wide grin.

The girls and I scouted thrift shops on Saturday mornings, and returned home in the afternoons with twenty-five cent paperback books one week, a thirty-five cent sugar bowl another week. A fifteen dollar wood bookshelf, used marble salt and pepper shakers, and more than anything a sense of home and family. The girls made a sign for our bathroom, "**THE LADIES ROOM**." All of our spirits began to rise.

But Andrew continued to slide.

"Where have you been?" I asked him one night during a rare phone call. "The girls need you."

"You should have thought of that before you walked out on me, Kath."

"If you had agreed to counseling, I wouldn't have walked out on you. And anyway, what happened to us? We always said that *we* would be different. That if we ever split up, we'd put the girls' needs first. And no matter what our feelings were for each other, we'd keep the lines of communication open."

"Well, that was easy to say *then*. But if we were so god damned capable of communicating right now, we wouldn't be separated in the first place."

"Andrew, it's the girls we're talking about. They need to see you."

Erupting in anger Andrew said, "Who do you think you are anyway? You spent three months having a fucking nervous breakdown—You're still off the deep end if you ask me. And now, because of you, I'm falling apart, and you're telling *me* about proper behavior?"

"Not proper behavior, Andrew. Just what's fair to the girls. Don't take your anger at me out on them."

"Why not? Who should I take my anger out on? I'm doing them a favor, believe me. Tell them I'm dead," and he hung up.

Days in Court: Vindication

"It won't take a detective for the jurors to figure this case out, Neil. I have a clean mental and physical medical history before the injection. They'll see that the nurse was working three jobs and was exhausted at the time of the injection. Plus, we won the arbitration, with the arbitrator saying the case was straightforward. Even though we only were awarded $33,000, that was before I was hospitalized or had substantial medical bills, and we didn't know the extent of my injury or its 'lifetime' prognosis then. And you yourself said that arbitration awards are generally low."

"We'll see, Kath. You must know I think your case is strong—I took it on contingency."

Neil lined up doctors—"expert witnesses"—willing to testify on my behalf as to my credibility and the extent of my injury, both mental and physical.

The trial couldn't be over soon enough. For years now I had been running into people on the street, in the grocery store, at the park, that would ask about my health and the status of my trial. It was embarrassing that so many people knew that I had been hospitalized in a psychiatric ward. Since my injury was not visible and so many doctors had denied it, I was sensitive about not being believed, and my time in a psych ward didn't help.

Winning my trial wouldn't alter my pain, but the vindication would prove both my pain and my sanity. And I looked forward to compensation, to paying my bills rather than juggling them, and to having the money to provide for physical therapy and the girls.

Throughout the preparation of my case, Neil followed the status of the Micra Act, a 1975 California law that attempted to curb the malpractice insurance crisis by limiting medical malpractice awards to "economic" damages plus a cap of $250,000 for pain and suffering. The Micra Act's constitutionality was under review in the California Supreme Court. If the Supreme Court upheld the limit as constitutional, Neil's potential fee—a percentage of my recovery—would be substantially limited, and Neil had already invested heavily in my case, both in time and money.

In February of 1985, over two years after we filed suit and one year before the trial, the Supreme Court upheld the Micra Act. Would Neil's priorities shift to other more lucrative cases?

As I read the newspaper accounts, I was sympathetic to the insurance crisis. I'd always read about people receiving large settlements, and they frequently struck me as way out of proportion to the actual damages. Now I was on the other end, and while a quarter of a million dollars sounded enormous, my entire future was an unknown at this point. Besides legal expenses, I was approaching my lifetime cap on medical insurance and was concerned how to obtain new insurance that would cover my pre-existing condition.

Because of the Micra Act cap, I questioned Neil whether there were other areas of recovery for me other than pain and suffering.

"Well," Neil said. "Loss of earning capacity is a consideration. But that's a tough one, because you never earned much. But you're young," he said. "You married early. You've been raising young children. It stands to reason you would have worked at some point. But I don't know, Kath," he said shaking his head.

Days in Court: Vilification

"There are no facts, only interpretations."

—Frederich Nietzsche

"That which does not kill you makes you stronger."

—Frederich Nietzsche

The defense never physically examined me. I waited all through the years preceding the trial for the defense to attempt to discover personally whether and how I was injured. The request never came.

I couldn't understand it.

Word did come, however, of an exam by a defense *psychiatrist.*

Dr. Payne, the psychiatrist, asked me to take yet another M.M.P.I., in his small empty waiting room. He then interviewed me for about forty minutes. He later testified that we spent three hours together.

He asked me a variety of questions, some more than once, and frequently stayed with the same question, asking me to think a little harder.

"Have you done any acting, Kathleen?"

"None that I can recall. I was shy growing up and I've certainly not done any as an adult."

"Ah, but you must have done some, Kathleen. We all do, school plays, etc."

"Well, I was in a play at a summer program at my elementary school when I was in fourth or fifth grade."

"And what part did you play?"

"I was the King."

"They had you play the part of the King. Why?"

"I don't know, I was probably one of the older kids."

Dr. Payne's notes: "She notes that it was 'exciting' for her to come to California as a young girl. She became active in theater classes at the YMCA and at her school. She indicates she was in at least 20 theatrical productions, and furthermore was 'usually the lead' during her summer playground theatrical experiences. (It is not unusual to have such a history of early dramatic training and propensity in people who show obvious histrionic and hysterical trends as adults.)"

"Have you ever had a needle administered other than the injection that you believe has created all these problems for you?"

"Oh well, I imagine I have," I said. "I had all of the appropriate immunizations as a child."

"What about as an adult?"

"Well probably, certainly I've had blood tests, that kind of thing."

"Any injections?"

"Well, let's see, I had one after Amanda was born — a routine injection to prevent excessive bleeding."

Dr. Payne's notes: "Following childbirth, she had a bleeding problem, remembers receiving various injections for medications —"

"What about your diet Kathleen? I see you requested a vegetarian diet while in the hospital."

"Well, that was more a reflection on the hospital food than dietary preference." I laughed. He didn't.

"Have you always been a vegetarian Kathleen?"

"I don't know what I am," I said, tired of questions.

Dr. Payne smiled and made a note to himself.

Whether or not I was a "vegetarian" I had no idea. I know some vegetarians eat no meat, I thought. And some no dairy products. I did eat some red meat growing up. Now, I thought, I rarely eat red meat, but I do eat fish, chicken and eggs. So what am I?

"Do you avoid milk and dairy products?"

"No, I eat a lot of dairy products with the exception of milk. I don't like milk. It makes me feel nauseated."

"Didn't you worry about calcium intake growing up?"

"I didn't, but my mother did. She discussed with a doctor my dietary preferences. He said they were fine, providing I took a calcium pill daily. Two years later I was diagnosed as having excess calcium deposits."

Dr. Payne's notes: "...and furthermore, associated with her being a 'vegetarian since I was a child', possible treatment for a B vitamin deficiency. At another time, as a youth in school, she had difficulties with 'calcium deposits' from 'not eating meat or drinking milk'."

When I later read Dr. Payne's notes, the misstatements about the bleeding problem and the possible B vitamin deficiency stood out. They came up again during the trial. As it turns out, vitamin B-12 deficiency occurs in some vegetarians and has symptoms which include a sore back, numbness and tingling, moodiness and delusions, and damage resulting to the central nervous system ultimately resulting in spinal deterioration.

The lack of a physical exam was part of the defense strategy. It allowed them to speculate throughout the trial about the nature and causes of my injury. Every symptom or diagnosis that could be presented to the jury would be an additional source of confusion, an additional reason for the jurors to question whether a negligent injection was the cause of my pain.

"Aren't these also symptoms of multiple sclerosis? Was she tested for this?"

Or anemia? Or diabetes mellitus? Or vitamin B-12 deficiency? Or alcohol consumption? Was she tested for each one of these?

Once the trial began there was a new defense attorney.

"Where's Millicent Browne?" I asked Neil.

"Who knows?" he said smiling. "Maybe they felt they had to call in their heavy artillery."

On the stand the defense attorney asked me, "So Kathleen, you stated that the doctor in the hospital emergency room on the night of the injection seemed hurried. You didn't like him from the start, did you?"

"It wasn't that I didn't like him as much as he seemed distracted and hurried and he didn't examine me."

"And you didn't like that, did you?"

"No, I guess not."

"And you wanted to punish him for treating you in this manner, didn't you?"

"What?" I asked. "I…"

The defense counsel cut me off.

"Kathleen, let me understand. Hadn't your pediatrician previously told you that Columbus Memorial was the 'one to call' in the case of an emergency?"

"Yes."

"And, isn't that in fact why you went to Columbus Memorial?"

"Yes."

"And yet when the doctor ordered an injection you were uncomfortable?"

"Well, yes. Dr. Kohn had advised me to avoid medicine while I was breast feeding."

"But in fact Dr. Kohn was the physician that recommended the hospital."

"Yes —"

"I fail to see the cause for concern, Kathleen. The hospital had been recommended. You were quite ill. You went to the hospital for help, did you not?"

"I did —"

"And when it was offered, or prescribed, you were nervous. You never liked the doctor on duty that night, did you?"

"Never liked him? I'd never seen him before. I didn't like it that he never examined me but ordered medication, and was unwilling to check with Dr. Kohn, as Dr. Kohn had always instructed me to do."

"Exactly. You didn't like him and you didn't trust him."

Meeting me one morning on our way into court, Neil was excited. "This is it," he said. "I've got it."

"What? What do you have?" I asked, eyeing the file in his hand.

"A case that helps our position regarding loss of earning capacity, Kath."

"What kind of case?" I asked, interested.

"We're in a hurry to get to court, Kathy, but here's the analogy: Imagine a couple has a grand piano, but they hadn't played it. Someone steals the piano. Does the insurance company reimburse them even though they hadn't played it yet?"

But I had married at eighteen and would be entering the working force in my early thirties—would the jurors be able to place value on my remaining fifty plus working years without a W-2 on the prior ten?

Why would I have filed a medical malpractice suit, other than for financial gain, the defense frequently suggested to the jurors.

"That's interesting you brought that up," Neil said one day in a cool, Columbo type fashion to Dr. Payne on the witness stand. "The possibility of financial gain is a pretty strong motivator for many people, isn't it?"

"For the majority of people, yes," Dr. Payne said authoritatively.

"Let's talk a little," Neil said calmly, "about your reasons for being here today."

Dr. Payne's expression changed slightly, and he was silent.

"Dr. Payne, who asked you here today?"

"Well, as a physician, reviewing Kathleen's records —"

"Dr. Payne, on who's behalf are you testifying today?"

"Well I —" Dr. Payne paused, then said nothing.

"Dr. Payne, are you being paid to appear here today?"

"Well yes."

"Who is writing that check?" And when Dr. Payne failed to answer, Neil continued. "Dr. Payne, is the defense paying you to appear here today?"

"Yes —"

"How much are they paying you?"

The defense attorney, Brad Martin, objected. Both attorneys approached the bench.

Neil argued. "We've heard, your honor, so often through this trial about financial gain. But in fact all of us have a reason for being here today and I think that it is relevant to determine why Dr. Payne is here, what in fact he has to gain from testifying."

"Objection overruled," the judge ordered, agreeing with Neil.

"Dr. Payne, you are being paid by the defense for testifying here today, are you not?"

"I am."

"And you have testified for the defense before, on other cases, have you not?"

"Objection," Brad Martin called out.

"Overruled."

"Yes," answered Dr. Payne.

"And in fact you hope to testify for them again, don't you? Dr. Payne, what are you being paid by the defense for testifying?"

"Well, including the time I met with Kathleen, the MMPI I administered, the medical records I reviewed, and my testimony in this trial —"

"Yes," said Neil, "what are you being paid for your time?"

"Ten thousand dollars."

An audible murmur could be heard from among the jurors. "Well, I guess all of us have motivating factors to be here today," Neil said with a grin spreading from ear to ear.

Daisy Racine, the nurse that had administered the injection and had shown up at the arbitration with cutoff jeans and a pink bow in her hair, arrived in court looking like she should be on the cover of "Working Woman" — a professional woman of the 80's. She had on a wool suit and pumps, and her hair pulled back off her face in a tight bun.

She spoke clearly and seriously. She could now easily answer all the questions she had trouble with at the arbitration.

Neil asked her if, as she had stated in the emergency room and confirmed at the arbitration, she had four boys, skied and worked three jobs.

"Yes," Nurse Racine said to all three counts.

He did not, however, ask her if it was true that on the night of the injection she had not slept in 72 hours.

"Why didn't you ask her that?" I berated him.

"Well, that was a judgment call Kathy. One of the first things you learn in law school is to never ask a witness a question unless you know you will get the answer you want."

"Oh come on Neil," I said impatiently. "The jurors would have realized there was something funny going on if she admitted everything I recalled from that night but this one statement, that is in fact an incriminating one."

"I wasn't so sure Kathleen," he said uneasily. "I wasn't so sure."

"If you deal with a fox, think of his tricks."

—Jean de la Fontaine

On two separate occasions, opposing counsel Brad Martin sat in the hall with one of his witnesses close to where the jurors were gathered just before court was to begin.

The first time, he pronounced forcefully to Dr. Shein that Lee Jones was a very young, inexperienced doctor who meant well, but hadn't a clue as to what was what, and that Dr. Jones had in fact seriously misindicated the sciatic notch on a chart the previous day.

Later that same day Dr. Shein, a specialist testifying on behalf of the defense, mismarked the sciatic notch in his testimony too. He missed it by more than Lee Jones had.

"This chart is in fact poorly drawn," Brad Martin objected in the courtroom.

Again in the corridor, with the jurors close by, Brad Martin initiated a conversation with Daisy Racine, the nurse that had administered the injection. Brad Martin said loudly "Can you believe this case made it here today? I mean for goodness sake, you teach a class on administering injections. If anybody knows injections, it's you!" and they both laughed.

I was furious and I told Neil.

"He did that?" Neil said, his face reddening.

"Yes," I said. "Tell the judge!"

Neil was quiet. "No," he said, "Brad knows that kind of thing isn't permitted. He must be feeling desperate to do something so transparent, and the jurors will be able to see right through that anyway."

On the witness stand, I was asked if anyone in my family ever had ulcers. I stated that my father and Andrew both had ulcers.

"Were you ever diagnosed as having ulcers, Kathleen?"

"No, never," I said firmly.

Dr. Payne was again put on the stand and questioned. He smiled and suggested that I was mentally ill, schizophrenic. So schizophrenic that I had no idea who had ulcers, that in fact it was me. The defense introduced into evidence records of my ulcers.

I was still reeling from the schizophrenic diagnosis, when Neil whispered angrily to me, "How could you keep this from me, Kath?"

"I never had ulcers," I nearly screamed. "And what is he talking about? Me, schizophrenic?"

"Kath, stop," Neil said, angry.

"I didn't keep anything from you Neil," I said to him at recess, my stomach knotting. "I've never had ulcers. Unless," I added sarcastically, "it was maybe my other personality."

"Oh Kathleen," he said removing his glasses and wiping his eyes. "If you never had ulcers then where did they get the medical records just submitted into evidence?"

"Neil, I have never been diagnosed as having ulcers in my life," I said shrilly. "There's been a mistake. What doctor is it?"

"Dr. Meade."

"Let me call him now," I said hurriedly.

"If you want to call him, go ahead Kathleen," Neil said looking beat.

I reached Dr. Meade on the phone. He was appalled. "Never!" he said surprised. " Someone came on behalf of the defense and copied both Andrew's records and yours. They must have mixed them up."

"Except that Neil said my name is all over them, and the sex indicated is female."

"They must have altered them," he said more quietly.

Altered them?

"Can you testify to that?" I asked, embarrassed to involve him, but feeling desperate.

"I would be happy to, Kathleen, but I am leaving immediately for an emergency in New York."

"I'm in trial now," I said desperately.

"I'm sorry, but I have to make this trip." He paused. "I'd be happy to testify when I return."

"Neil we need to delay the trial," I said feeling both guilty and relieved that Dr. Meade said he'd testify. I'd grown quite aware of how undesirable it was for members of the medical profession to testify against members of their own profession.

"We can't delay the trial," Neil said impatiently, in a tone implying this was a ludicrous thought.

"Why? I want the jurors to know not only that I don't have ulcers, but also that someone altered the records."

"Trust me Kathy, we just can't. Now we have other things to be working on, will you stop talking about this and give me a minute to think?"

So now my medical records contained "ulcers," and the jurors thought me schizo, and I was confused. Did Neil believe me? I wondered. This wasn't a time when I could deal with my own attorney doubting me.

The defense consistently put witnesses on the stand who made "slips" that were false but, I could only imagine, made considerable impressions on the jury.

The jurors had no way of knowing these things were lies; to them they must have represented "secrets."

The defense attorney asked Nurse Racine if in fact she wouldn't have taken the task of administering an injection seriously being a single mother, since if she did her job poorly she would lose her job and she wouldn't be able to support her kids.

"Objection!" Neil approached the bench. "That was totally uncalled for. Nurse Racine's continued employment will not be based on the outcome of this trial. For defense counsel to imply this is extremely prejudicial to my client. Your honor must specifically inform the jury that Nurse Racine's job is not in question."

"Strike from the record," said the judge. "The jury shall ignore this line of questioning."

In addition it was agreed that my TMJ that had been diagnosed after the discovery cutoff would be off limits during the trial. TMJ (temporo mandibular joint disorder), which had resulted from my gritting and grinding my teeth from stress, caused headaches and facial pain.

We carefully deleted it from my testimony regarding pain management treatments.

Dr. Payne, on the stand, made reference to a visit at the pain clinic where I "presented" myself claiming an earache, jaw pain, difficulty eating solid foods and a severe headache. "This is clearly a patient whose complaints know no limit," he said.

"Objection!" called Neil.

At the bench again, Neil told the judge, "Defense counsel knows that Kathleen had TMJ diagnosed after the discovery cutoff, and that we claim it was caused by her injury. Counsel requested that, to avoid delaying the trial further, it not be brought up in court. Now counsel has used that agreement to prejudice the jury against my client, to make it appear she had unfounded complaints and is a hypochondriac."

"Strike from the record," said the judge.

One more secret, the jurors must have thought.

Neil's closing argument was brilliant.

He summarized my life and reviewed my clear medical history prior to the injection. He reminded the jurors that the defense had admitted belief in my pain, and had only questioned the cause.

"The defense has speculated on possible reasons for Kathleen's pain. Vegetarianism, four months of alcohol consumption, even wearing tight jeans. I submit that the defense tried to distract you from the most probable cause — the negligent injection of Phenergan on the night her pain began in the emergency room of Columbus Memorial Hospital."

He discussed motivational factors, reminding the jurors of Dr. Payne's ten thousand dollar fee.

He spoke about pain. "All of us have experienced pain at some time. Think back on your worst pain. Imagine it was due to someone else's negligence, and that it would never go away. Well that's what Kathleen has to live with. Every day. For the rest of her life. Because of the negligence of a nurse who had not slept in 72 hours, and a hospital who failed to supervise her."

The jurors listened intently, obviously moved. I warmed at the thought that Neil had slipped in to the closing argument the fact that Nurse Racine had not slept in 72 hours, although I still wished he'd questioned her about it.

He touched on the difficulty of remembering pain. "You know they say," he said smiling, "if pain could be remembered, all families would be limited to one child."

He was eloquent, and I knew I'd won.

Day in Court: Verdict

"That psychiatrist just *lied*," I said angrily, tearfully describing my experience in court to Marie, an old friend married to an attorney. "Well of course he did," Marie said. "Didn't you know he would? Didn't your attorney tell you he would?"

"How could Neil have *known* he was going to lie?"

"Because that's what he was hired for, Kathy — do you remember Roland? You've met him at my house for parties on a number of occasions. He's a defense psychiatrist too — an expert witness. He's given a profile of what he needs to 'find' before the patient ever enters his office. He's paid to find what the defense wants him to find."

"Oh my god," I said, feeling sick. "Marie, is that the way our court system works?"

"Sometimes, Kathy. And your attorney should have told you," she said tenderly.

"But we are talking about a court of justice," said the renowned New York judge Learned Hand to his colleague, Justice Oliver Wendell Holmes, Jr.

"No," replied Justice Holmes, "it is only a court of law."

All of the evidence had been presented. The closing arguments were completed, one week after the trial began. On a Thursday afternoon, the jurors received a list of ten written questions to consider, and they filed out of the courtroom to go home.

Friday was an off day.

Saturday and Sunday passed.

Monday was President's Day.

The wait was awful.

The following week the jury deliberated. And deliberated. And then they filed back into the courtroom, ready to announce their decision.

"Question 1," the foreman read. "was the defendant negligent in the hospital care and treatment of plaintiff? Finding — No."

No, the defendant was not negligent, I repeated to myself.

Based upon this finding, the remaining questions were irrelevant.

That was it. It's over, I thought.

I waited for some emotion to sweep over me — anger, depression, anything. I was numb.

The judge then asked the jury if they would be so kind as to step into his chambers so that he could thank them individually and so that the counsel could speak with them briefly.

Neil turned to me and said that I could go home, that he wanted to ask the jurors a few questions.

I stood up numb.

I remember thanking the jurors quietly and nodding my head in the direction of the two jurors Neil had said held out in my favor up until the last minute.

Then I drove home.

The next morning I called Neil. "Thank you for representing me, Neil. I wish the outcome had been different, but I wouldn't have wanted to be in that courtroom with anyone different."

"It's good to hear you say that Kathy."

"What about appealing the case?"

"I'm not an appellate attorney, Kath," Neil said. "Anyway, you have no basis for an appeal. An appeal is based upon a misreading of the law, not the facts. And the transcript alone from the trial would cost thousands of dollars."

He was silent.

"What did the jurors say, Neil? Why did they rule against me?"

"I don't know," he said. "They voiced several concerns. Even our own doctors couldn't agree on the exact injection site and the precise diagnosis of the injury. In addition, one of your first treating physicians, Dr. Christian, wrote that 'a nerve branch was *inadvertently* irritated by the injection.' "

"The jurors asked why I asked the nurse about 3 jobs, skiing, 4 boys, but not about not having slept in 72 hours. Ultimately, they weren't sure who to believe and in the absence of a belief one way or the other, they had to rule against us."

Recovery

"Illness is in part what the world has done to a victim, but in larger part it is what the victim has done with his world, and with himself."

—Karl Menninger

The trial was over, as was my marriage. I had no idea what to do. "I'll tell you what to do," Andrew said on the phone. "Come back to me. You'll have medical insurance, the girls will have a father and financially you won't have to worry."

"We can't go back, Andrew," I said heavily. I wish we could, I thought, wondering what our futures held. I was overwhelmed by guilt for the toll this had taken on all of our lives. But we had passed turning back.

People generally met the outcome of my trial with astonishment. What kind of attorney did you have? they would ask. How could you have lost? I had nothing left in me, not enough anyway to answer them intelligently. I didn't know how to condense the last four years into a brief casual conversation nor did I have the desire to.

Neil had advised me through the years preceding the trial, that given the opportunity, we should settle the case out of court. But the opportunity for any more than the arbitration award never arose.

Once in court however, I was confident.

Neil, knowing this, was uneasy. "Once you get in front of twelve jurors, all bets are off," he cautioned. "You can never be sure of what will happen in court."

Not believing Neil, I needed to find out for myself. And now I can only echo his sentiment.

I've been asked, and I've asked myself, whether Neil was the right attorney for this case. I guess the only flaw Neil had was integrity. He didn't want to win this case whatever the cost. Nor did I.

Neil referred me to Dr. Daniels, hoping he would help my pain, knowing he would refuse to testify. He accepted my admission to the psych ward, knowing the negative impact it would have on my case. And he visited me there saying, "It's not so bad Kathy. It's like a college dorm." He accepted my leaving Andrew five months before the case came to trial, realizing that it crumbled the "high school sweetheart" picture he had hoped to paint.

I know the Micra Act's effective limitation on attorney's fees placed Neil at a significant disadvantage to the defense, who had no such limit on their fees and resources.

And I came to understand that win or lose, the cost of a trial was incredibly high. The cost, when I was already in chronic pain, of having every area of my past and present life turned inside out and made hash of in front of twelve strangers and me.

So now where was I?

"Kathleen, you need to put all this behind you. Start fresh. Move on."

Good idea, I would think. How do I do that?

"Let go. It's not helping anyone, especially you, that you're so angry. If you keep this up you'll make yourself sick."

"Kathleen, anger turns people off. You'll never be able to start over if you carry this thing with you."

What the hell should I feel? I wondered. How can I not feel angry? "Move on," echoed in my ears. To where? I thought, exhausted. Where should I move on to?

I couldn't seem to forget. And as much as I didn't want to, I carried with me everywhere a constant, vivid reminder. Pain.

I knew that I needed to make a living, to be guarded with my health, and to make up for lost time with the girls. I thought of a variety of things to take on to make money, and to have flexible hours as both the girls and my shaky health required. But I also knew that I wanted to enjoy what I was doing and to feel productive. Any energy I had for stress, or negative factors, or unpleasantness was used up by pain. I didn't have a natural reserve available to help me cope with a miserable job.

How could I care for the girls, obtain medical insurance — which I'd be losing when the divorce became final — and not risk ruining my physical and emotional health. I sat with the Sunday classified ads and a pot of coffee, determined to find something.

I took a job as a receptionist at a law firm. My first week, telling one of the attorneys about what a liar Dr. Payne had been, and how surprised and disheartened I'd become about the system, I said, "My court case was like a circus."

"I'm sure it was, Kathleen," he said. "I always liken court to Las Vegas."

"Yeah, I always thought justice was served. But I guess it's all a gamble."

"The only likeness isn't the gambling," he said dryly. "Court is sadly enough full of prostitutes, too — 'experts' willing to testify to anything for a price."

"In proportion as he simplifies his life, the laws of the universe will appear less complex, and solitude will not be solitude, nor poverty poverty, nor weakness weakness. If you have built castles in the air, your work need not be lost; that is where they should be. Now put the foundations under them."

—*Henry David Thoreau,* Walden

My job as a receptionist answered my medical insurance problem, provided a small income, and allowed me to leave it behind when I went home at night.

On Friday nights I'd buy "goodies" at the store and the girls and I would snuggle up on their futon, watching television and reading. Those nights I would sleep twelve hours and this was my salvation. I was exhausted, physically, emotionally, and financially.

Without my mother, I couldn't have done it. She picked the girls up after school three nights out of five, and cooked them dinner as often. She bought them clothes and school supplies and attended the girls' school functions with me or in place of me. She baked pies with them and played beauty parlor and planted flowers. She told them stories about childhood, hers, mine and theirs. She provided continuity, and fun and love in abundance.

I left the house at 7 a.m. and arrived no sooner than twelve hours later, after work and physical therapy. The girls had an equally long day and I'd sometimes wonder if this was all fair to them. There we go again, fair, I thought frustrated. I couldn't say that it was fair, and I didn't want to say in a resigned fashion, "That's life," so instead I said, "This is right now. We won't always live this way. It's temporary." That made us all feel better.

I could see a better life out there and I wanted it. Between working, trying to spend time with the girls, and turning our apartment into a home, I began to feel incredibly run down. I thought back on some of what I'd learned at the pain clinic. They had said that I needed to accept the fact that I was not the person that I had been, and that I would never be. That my stamina, my outlook, my stress level, my general health, would never be the same. And that if I recognized this and operated within reasonable boundaries, I would fare better. I hated "reasonable boundaries."

At the pain clinic, they said the average person has the energy for the little stresses that occur daily. Traffic jams, long lines, a forgotten appointment, the flu. But a person in chronic pain uses up their energy dealing with pain. Therefore it is extremely important that a person suffering from chronic pain reduce, to the best of their ability, their everyday stresses. Shop when stores aren't crowded, avoid hours when traffic is likely to be at its worst, attend only those social functions likely to be enjoyed, not those that are an "obligation." Eat a balanced diet, avoid alcohol, sleep regularly, exercise. Stop and smell the roses. Things that anyone would benefit from, but things that someone with the stress of daily pain must do.

Providing for the girls presently and in the future was of grave concern to me. The chemical imbalance I'd suffered from still terrified me.

"How do I know that won't happen to me again?" I asked Dr. Jones weakly. "I don't have it in me to go through that again. I remember being locked up feeling my skin crawl. I..."

He interrupted me, "Kathleen, there are no guarantees, but I would be very surprised if you ever go through anything like that again."

I'm surprised I ever went through anything like that at all, I thought shaking.

The girls had the same concern. If I coughed, they came running. Are you all right, mommy? Are you sick? Do you have to go to the doctors? Do you have to go into the hospital?

Dr. Jones transferred to New York in June, 1987 and I missed him terribly. I remembered how dark everything had been when I'd met him. And how resistant I'd been to "sitting around talking about things we can't do anything about." Strangely enough I found that sitting around talking about how angry I felt *was* helpful. I remember that for months after meeting Dr. Jones, whenever he would approach my feelings for the nurse that administered the injection, I intellectualized my feelings.

"You must be angry, Kathleen," Dr. Jones would say.

"No," I would say blandly, "not really. I mean she didn't intend to do it."

"Well, how about the doctors that wouldn't help because they didn't want to get involved?"

"Well, you can't blame them," I would say. "I mean they had practices to maintain and probably families to take care of. The American Medical Association is powerful and would certainly frown upon treating a patient involved in a medical malpractice case."

"Kathleen," Dr. Jones would say, leaning towards me, "I'm not asking you what your head is telling you, or what's fair, or what's right. I'm asking you what you are *feeling*."

"We should set them all on fire," I said one day, in the same monotone. His face lit up like the Fourth of July.

"What?" he asked smiling. "Can you repeat that?"

"I hate them all," I said almost choking on the words.

"Good for you," he said leaning back in his chair.

It was amazing to me how angry I was and how much venom I spilled.

“I’ve got to tell you something,” I said to Dr. Jones one day after I’d spent about a half hour insulting the world. “What we are doing here is the opposite of everything my mother ever taught me. How this will be helpful is beyond me.”

“It will be Kathleen, I promise. While you have a chemical imbalance and need medication, you are also terribly angry. Your depression stems from your anger. It’s the knife turned inward.”

It was amazing how helpful it was. I began to feel an incredible release as the angry, hurt, self pitying words spilled out of me session after session.

“It’s great, isn’t it?” my girlfriend Mary said once. “I mean,” she continued, “You go in with a wheelbarrow full of troubles and dump them all on your shrink’s floor, and when you leave … you leave them there.”

It still strikes me as amazing that talking about pain, a pain that no one could alleviate, would prove to be so helpful.

“All that garbage has to go somewhere Kathleen,” Dr. Jones said. “It’s better out in the open than inside. That’s the stuff ulcers are made of. ”

When I was suffering from the chemical imbalance nothing mattered. I knew that it should, and on some level I wanted it to, but it didn’t. An enormous shadow had been cast over everything. I felt there was no reason to get up, and nothing held any interest or joy. I had no attention span, was easily confused and perpetually exhausted.

“How does your depression differ from sadness?” Dr. Jones asked me.

“If someone dies, you generally think back on the wonderful times you shared. That’s what makes their absence so painful, so sad. Sadness leads you to hold loved ones closer, heightens your senses, makes you painfully aware of the passage of time. Sadness is grey, maybe with the color of anger, of grief, of fear. But depression is black—a combination of the loss of all memories other than dark ones and the loss of all hope for the future. Depression is like being in hell with no hope of leaving and no memory of ever having been anywhere different.”

When I asked to have the chemical imbalance explained to me, Dr. Jones said, “Well, we’re not sure whether your brain has stopped producing a necessary chemical or whether the chemical can’t get from point A to point B.”

I was conscious of the fact that only a weak, crazy, evil mother would consider committing suicide . And that only helped further the feeling that everyone would be better off without me.

"It is hopelessness even more than pain that crushes the soul."

—William Styron

As I began to mend, Dr. Jones represented hope to me, as did each new treatment I would try or doctor I would see. I needed to believe that I was not going to spend my life in this kind of pain. That there was some treatment not yet known to me, or that research was being done. I needed an element of hope for my sanity. And now Dr. Jones was in New York.

Not only was Dr. Jones gone, but I was also feeling the loss of Dr. Rosenblatt's acupuncture treatments, which had fallen victim to financial constraints and geographic limits imposed by my new job and Los Angeles freeways. I had been skeptical and terrified of acupuncture at first, but I quickly changed my mind. Acupuncture was the first treatment to significantly reduce my stress and pain without significant "side" effects. Even in my poor health, I felt a sense of serenity and peace after each visit. I sorely missed both the treatments and Dr. Rosenblatt's gentle manner.

It had been suggested to me many times that I see a chiropractor. This never made sense to me for two reasons. First, my back was not the problem. It was a nerve injury with resulting muscle cramping. My back was fine, and although intellectually I had no problem with chiropractors, my gut screamed *charlatan*.

But once again, with the injection site continuing to burn and cramp, my head throbbing, my leg numb and tingly, I was willing to try almost anything.

"Doctor shopper," they'd called me in court. "When she doesn't like what one doctor says, she sees another and another. She's hoping to find one that will say what she wants to hear. And if she doesn't like what they say, she tries a new one."

And they were right. I was determined to find one that didn't predict a lifetime of pain for me. One that could help.

I made an appointment to see Dr. Bruce Oppenheim. His office was not only five minutes from my house, but he was open week-nights and weekends, and he was covered by my medical plan. X-rays and a medical history were taken and an appointment was made for me to return days later, so that Dr. Oppenheim, whom I had not yet met, would have a chance to review them with me.

As soon as I met Dr. Oppenheim, I liked him. "Well, you've certainly been through a lot," he said as he stepped into my exam room, my file and case history in his hand.

"Do you think you can help?" I asked. "I've already been through the U.C.L.A. Pain Clinic."

"Never mind them," he said smiling, exuding warmth and calm. "We'll be your pain clinic from now on."

I thought in the car on the way home of something Neil had said to me, after meeting both Dr. Jones and Dr. Rosenblatt.

"You sure know how to pick handsome doctors, Kath." I'd done it again, I thought, smiling to myself.

Why do you like Dr. Oppenheim so much? co-workers asked.

"Because he seems warm and caring and I trust him."

"Really? Will his 'warmness' help your nerve injury?"

I was shown a film on chiropractics and treatments began. Heat pads; tens unit, to which I still had a negative reaction; neck collar; and the orthostatic "rolling" table.

I remember the first time one of Dr. Oppenheim's assistants instructed me to hop up on the rolling table. It was a hard cot with a lump that moved up and down my spine, like a bakery rolling pin.

"I don't like that table," I said. "It doesn't help me,"

"How do you know? Come on, it will do you good."

"No, I don't like that table," I repeated. I was remembering Dr. Alexander, alias Marcus Welby. I used that table at his office. It had been unhelpful, painful, time consuming and costly.

"Dr. Oppenheim has prescribed this therapy for you, Kathleen. He wants you to use it."

"No," I said backing up. "You know when I'll get on that table?" I said icily.

"When?" he asked cheerfully.

"When hell freezes over."

A month went by. I felt about the same physically. Emotionally I felt hopeful however, like someone waiting for a package in the mail. Coming home from Dr. Oppenheim one evening, I had a funny sensation in my leg. I touched it, and my touch felt somewhat normal.

"I can feel my leg," I screamed. "Girls! Amanda and Acasia!" I screamed.

They came running. "Touch my leg," I said excited. They stared at me wide eyed, accustomed to hearing, don't touch my leg, be careful of my leg. Laughing, I said, "Go ahead. Touch mommy's leg."

They did so timidly.

"I felt that," I said excited. I began to cry.

My mom came in from the kitchen.

"I can feel my leg," I kept repeating. And then I couldn't feel it. My self controlled calm returned. How could I have been so foolish as to get my hopes up?

My mom hugged me tight. "You're tired honey. Otherwise you'd be able to see what a good sign this is. Believe me, it will get better. You'll get better. It's a wonderful sign that your leg felt normal for any period of time, no matter how brief."

I continued seeing Dr. Oppenheim and continued to have brief periods of feeling shortly afterwards, followed by periods of more intense pain. Dr. Oppenheim didn't seem to doubt that this was a good sign, but said that it would take time, and since I trusted him, I kept going.

My visits to Dr. Oppenheim were time consuming — the rolling table was now a standard part of my treatment — and I had very little time. But he inspired me. He'd enter each patient's room, full of life, as though they were the only person in the whole world.

"How are you doing?" he'd ask, and wait for an answer.

"Tired," I'd say, feeling the underdog. He'd laugh. "Gee, I wonder why," he'd continue, "You're working full time, raising two daughters, and coming here. But it will get better Kathleen. I see you as the type of person that will make it get better."

I'd arrive at his office at the end of the day, exhausted and unhappy and I'd leave feeling relaxed and hopeful.

"You'll lick this," he would say assuredly. "I can tell."

The chiropractic treatments were unable, and were never expected to, reduce the original pain from the injection. But they lessened the numbness and tingling in my left leg, the TMJ, headaches, and overall feeling of tension. In addition, through new x-rays, Dr. Oppenheim detected pinched nerves.

Pinched nerves? That was a new diagnosis.

"Probably as a result of compensating, Kathleen. You've altered your walking and sitting, and put additional pressure on your right leg."

Additional pressure? I was re-heeling my right shoe about once a month. That was, I now realized, a contributing factor as to why I felt the pain was increasing all these years. It was—notwithstanding the suggestions at the pain clinic that the pain was not increasing but my tolerance of the pain was decreasing.

Once again I was reminded that a person in chronic pain must clean up and improve those areas of his life, both emotional and physical, over which he has control, like a blind person who compensates by heightening his other senses.

As a result of Dr. Oppenheim's treatments, I found myself more able to cope. And more hopeful of new therapies and treatments.

"Dr. Oppenheim," I said one afternoon smiling , "you are one of three most wonderful men in my life."

"Thank you," he said smiling. "But now I guess what I want to know is, who are the other two?"

"Opportunity is missed by most people because it is dressed in overalls and looks like work."

—Thomas Edison

It was a slow recovery. For a few minutes, and then half an hour, and then more and more, I began to feel good. The whole world looked brighter during these times. And then the darkness would seep in. It was disappointing each time the brightness would begin to fade. I began to wonder which was real life. I began to wonder if I was manic depressive. I remembered patients in the psych ward with horrible mood swings and I wondered if that was my problem.

I thought back on Dr. Jones telling me how he saw me coming out of the deep depression I was in. He said the depression would lift a little and I would catch glimpses of something better. He said the glimpses would come more and more frequently, and last a little longer each time. And slowly, very slowly, the scale would tip and the good times would outweigh the bad. Until one day I would actually feel happy much of the time. And when I wasn't feeling happy I would have the clear perspective to know the bad mood was just that, and that it wouldn't last.

Maybe that was what was happening I thought. Maybe rather than my having a new problem, or diagnosis, I was actually improving.

It began to take less and less energy to do the mundane things in life. And I began to find that the "mundane" things could lose that quality with little effort on my behalf.

I began including one special thing in each day. A cup of cappuccino purchased on the way to work. A new paperback book. A chocolate croissant. Some daisies. Time and finances were tight, but I reminded myself of Brent holding up the smokehouse almonds in the psychiatric ward saying, "It's the little things in life."

"I am wealthy in my friends."

— *William Shakespeare*

Being a friend to someone in pain has to be generally unrewarding. Friendship with me had become mostly a one way street; I had little time, money or emotion to give at this point in my life. I remember canceling out on people or just plain turning down invitations far more than I ever accepted them. I never knew how I was going to feel at the actual time of a party or whatever. Embarrassed at canceling repeatedly, I finally just stopped accepting.

At the pain clinic, I'd overhear the family members and friends of patients say, "I want to help. I just don't know what to do. Tell me what to do." No way could I have told someone something helpful to do. But looking back, the answer was *any* gesture that indicates that someone truly cares is helpful.

From grand gestures to small, old friends found continual ways to help. And when I stopped believing in myself, they didn't. I was touched that they stuck by me, and amazed that new friends popped up to help me, people that I shared no past with, no history of give and take. And while the impact of their friendship must have been invisible to them at the time, their friendship brought to my dark days a sense of normalcy and sanity and even magic that made the present bearable and the future thinkable.

Carla Itkin, a friend since junior high, was always there for me and the girls. She watched Acasia and Amanda for a month of my hospitalization, the month before she got married, in the midst of sewing her wedding dress and organizing her wedding.

When I left Andrew she helped paint my apartment, and sewed lace curtains and beautiful floor pillows for it. She remembered every holiday for the girls, bringing them Valentine gifts, and Easter baskets, and sewing them gingham aprons and baking cookies with them at Christmas.

She invited me out constantly, knowing that ninety-nine percent of the time I wouldn't go. "Well, there's always that minute chance you'll say yes, isn't there Kathy?" she'd say good naturedly. "I'll probably have better luck next time … and don't think there won't be a next time, Kathy."

"Carla, why do you bother?" I'd ask amazed, exhausted and embarrassed.

"Bother? It's no bother. And anyway, don't forget, I remember all the fun we had and it's not just history Kathy. You won't always be so down and so stressed, and so I'll just wait. I've got time."

A few nights after I lost the lawsuit she called. "O.K.", she said, "I've given you a few days to hole up. Now you feel like some company?"

"No, thanks, Carla," I said appreciative, but desirous of hanging up and pulling the covers back over my head.

"I could bring good coffee," she said temptingly.

"No, the girls are asleep," I said without expression. "I'm going to do the same."

"I could bring Pepperidge Farm cookies — the Paris Collection."

"No, sounds good Carla, but not tonight," I said stubbornly.

"I could bring a Vogue magazine…"

"No, not tonight Carla, but thanks."

"And we could cut down all the models like we used to," she continued.

I found myself smiling. "O.K. Carla, I would love you to come over."

And later that night with cookies and coffee and Carla and Vogue magazine, I found myself laughing and wondering what I'd done to deserve such a faithful friend, as I looked at Carla stretched out on my living room floor, animatedly saying, "And look at this girl, Kathy. Talk about eyebrows! I mean what has she done to herself?" And on and on.

Sheila Lavery, the friend who had suggested the U.C.L.A. pain clinic, said over the phone one night, "Kathy, Michael and I were talking. You remember our little red Datsun?"

"Yeah," I said slowly.

"I know you love that '63 Dodge you have, Kathy, but how long can it last? And how safe can it be? The Datsun's a great car. Low mileage, runs like a charm. We've just used it for au pairs — anyway, we'd like you to have it."

"Have it?" I repeated, dumfounded.

"*Have* it," she echoed. "It would really make us happy, Kath, if you'd let us do this for you."

"But Sheila, you have four little girls. If nothing else, you could put the money away for college, or —"

"Kathy," she said firmly, "we want to do this. Say yes," she pleaded happily. "Just say yes."

Sheila called every night of my trial to see if I was o.k. She sent me flowers midway through the trial with a card that read, "With profound admiration."

She and Michael invited the girls and me over to all of her parties just as she had previously even though I was now the only single parent. We'd always had Easter brunch and an egg hunt at one of our houses for the girls, my two and her four. The week before the first Easter the girls and I were living in the apartment she called and asked when would be a good time for the brunch. "You mean you still want to do it?" I asked touched and surprised.

"Well, why wouldn't I?" she asked sounding genuinely confused.

"Well I thought it would be awkward ."

"Awkward? The only awkward thing would be explaining to Michael and the girls where you were if you didn't come."

Acasia best described Wira Daniels years ago, when I overheard her saying to a friend, "I don't need a fairy godmother. I have Auntie Wira." It was so easy for the girls' spirit of childhood to be swept away by the constant demands of my chronic pain and the accompanying financial and emotional pressures. Wira knew this and provided countless surprises and treasures, and a real sense of magic for the girls, while providing a constant stream of support for me as well. Wira bought us presents, took us out to eat, and cooked wonderful dinners for us. She took the girls shopping, out for ice cream, and swimming in her pool. In short, Wira was always thinking of us.

She and her husband, Tommy, welcomed us into their home and their hearts, and offered a sense of stability and constancy and support that we very much needed and grasped onto gratefully.

Mary Noordhof, a friend from Hollywood High, supported me with her intelligence and sense of humor. During her darkest moments she cannot suppress her love of life. She too lives with chronic pain and, over coffee, automatically and without thinking, we'd find ourselves offering Tylenol to each other.

"Want one?"

"Not now thanks, just had some," or "Oh yes, I'd love two."

"They're not candy you know," Carla said laughing once after observing this.

"Nope, they're better!" we chimed in unison.

Albert Schweitzer said that there is a "fellowship of those who bear the mark of pain." Mary was my "fellow." She lives with pain and lives to laugh. She advised and supported and commiserated with me, regarding pain and my frequent disappointment with our legal and medical systems. Along the way, she could always bring a smile, if not to my face, to my heart.

Mark Iungerich, who owned a local auto repair shop, continually serviced my car for what I am sure was a fraction of the actual cost, and met me on the San Diego Freeway once during rush hour when I was having car problems. He put all new tires on my car once when I had left it in for a routine tune up. "The tires are on me Kath. I hated seeing you and the girls drive around with those old ones."

I looked around at his auto shop, "HI Quality Motors," and at my 1963 Dodge, in stark contrast to the Mercedes and BMW's in his lot.

"Why did you do this?" I asked stunned, on the verge of tears.

"Well, I know if I hang on to you as a customer long enough you'll get one of these," he said laughing, pointing to a gorgeous convertible Mercedes in his lot.

When I moved out with the girls I was terrified. I'd never lived alone and now I was solely responsible for the girls. If there was a noise in the night, or a spider in the bathroom, or an earthquake, I was now the responsible adult. Kathy and John Gleason, my downstairs neighbors, assured me repeatedly that they were there for me anytime I needed them.

If I felt lonely and wanted to talk they would make the girls popcorn or give them cookies and sit and talk with me. If I was exhausted or stressed out and needed time to myself, they understood that, too.

Shortly after moving in, my refrigerator broke. I had no money and didn't know what to do. "I'll tell you what to do," John said. "Pick out a new refrigerator, and we'll pay for it. You can make small payments to us whenever you have a few dollars."

On Easter, they left two Easter baskets at our back door.

Frequently there would be a knock at the back door, and when I'd answer it there would be no one there, but a surprise … nuts, candy, fruit.

And they offered continual encouragement. "It will get better Kathleen," Kathy would say, seeing me in the laundry room , or carrying in bundles late at night, looking worn. "We've all had our dark time Kathleen. It passes. I promise." And, strangely, I believed her.

And then my mother. For years, through all of this, she'd come over, bringing homemade pie or stew or brownies, and flowers and magazines. She would talk for as long or as little as I liked. She would do laundry and dishes and vacuum and sweep. I remember days where I felt incapable of speaking but in which I derived enormous comfort in her presence, in hearing the mundane sounds of a normal household. I remember wanting to let her know how much it meant to me, and not knowing how, and being fearful that she wouldn't know, that she would think her visits and her household help went unnoticed. But each time she was leaving, she would sit next to me, and stroke my hair, and say, "I love you Kathy. I'll be back tomorrow." And I would breathe an invisible sigh of relief.

When the girls were little, their favorite bedtime book was "GO DOG GO!"

I remember reading it to them night after night and often repeatedly during the same night.

"Why don't we pick a different book?" I'd ask.

"NO!" they would say in unison firmly.

They would mouth the words the entire time I read, and would derive obvious comfort from the familiar, the known.

When I became sick, I remember saying to my mother every day at the end of her visit, just as she was about to leave —

"Was I ever any different? Any fun?"

Never once did she say, "Honey you ask me that every day." Never once did she seem annoyed or exhausted by the question. Each time she responded as though it was an entirely new and altogether interesting thought.

"Were you ever fun?" she'd repeat animatedly. "Why I remember the time..."

"The secret of being miserable is to have the leisure to bother about whether you are happy or not."

- George Bernard Shaw

A year after the trial and five years after the injection: I began to believe in myself and in life. I would set the alarm for five a.m. instead of five thirty, just so that I could savor a cup of coffee and listen to music.

My apartment felt like home and we felt like family. We weren't a family in the traditional way that we had been. It was different. And at times bittersweet.

I missed having someone I could turn to and say, "Aren't the girls beautiful? Incredible? A gift from heaven?"

I missed being special to someone.

And I felt responsible. What if something happens to me? I worried. The girls deserve better.

And what about a man? friends would ask. Isn't there a special someone in your life? Other than the girls?

I don't have time for a man, I would say, fully believing this. And I wasn't alone. I had the girls. Just having them asleep in the next room gave me a sense of life and a reason to be.

"Just wait until they grow up," Mary would say. "You'll be lonely. And they'll feel guilty and pressured if they're your whole life."

"Look, I have a full time job, two children, and chronic pain. I'm in debt up to my ears. I have no time or energy, and little interest in a man. And anyway, I'm not exactly a prize at this point. But I'm working on it," I'd add smiling.

Full Circle

"The tragedy of life is not that we die, but rather what dies inside a man while he lives."

—Albert Schweitzer

"I may go through the woods but I come out the other end."

—Mary Cartwright

I envisioned living in my tiny apartment, broke, for years. I knew no one would want any part of the life I was living, and I felt I had to come full circle to be a worthwhile half of a relationship. I wanted to set myself straight financially, reduce my pain level and raise my daughters. I knew I had nothing to give beyond that.

In 1987 I was sitting at my receptionist's desk and off the elevator stepped a memorable sight. A man in a business suit, about thirty years old, carrying a brief case, an over the shoulder bag, and a guitar. There was a wooden giraffe's head sticking out of his bag. He had curly black hair, a huge smile, and eyes that were alive and sensitive. He was there to see Mark Drooks, one of the attorneys in the firm. They were old friends and he was going to stay with Mark for a few days, while he was in California on business. He interested me.

Randy looked like he had a secret all the time. And I wanted in on the secret.

I had neither the time nor the inclination to get involved. But he was an attorney in Washington D.C. so I wasn't concerned about a serious, time consuming relationship. How much time could someone spare that lived three thousand miles away and had a demanding career?

Randy found time.

He sent me flowers, he sent the girls gifts. He flew out one weekend to work in a booth at the girls' school fair. He wrote us letters daily, as well as calling. For my birthday present in September 1987 he gave me a plane ticket to D.C.

It was fall, the leaves were changing, the air was crisp and we had a wonderful time.

"Look at this great elementary school," Randy said one evening as we walked his dog, Laika. "Would you consider moving Kathleen? I have extra rooms here and …"

"No, I wouldn't Randy," I interrupted.

"You wouldn't?" he asked seeming surprised, eyebrows raised.

"My life might look kind of disheveled to you. A single mom, working as a receptionist, driving an old beat up car and living in a one bedroom apartment with no furniture. But you know what's ironic? I've worked my ass off to get here. I'm just getting back on track, Randy. The girls and I aren't up for one more upheaval, even a positive one. And the three of us are very attached to my mom. We can't move."

"Well, I guess this is it," Randy said quietly at the airport.

"I guess so," I said realizing that we were falling in love. "The timing is all off, Randy. I have no room in my life for anyone right now, and my life is complicated. If I had it all together maybe things would be different,"

"Maybe," he said softly.

It was exhausting to try to rebuild my life. I had to start over financially and accept that while my old circle of friends were planning vacations and adding rooms and pools to their homes, I was shopping at thrift shops. I wasn't even close to looking *forward* financially; I was still paying for my past, and the daily mail continued to bring old medical bills to remind me.

Andrew was having a hard time, too.

"So, you glad you left Kath? Is it everything you'd hoped?"

"It's nothing yet Andrew, but I'll get there. So will you."

"With no help from you Kathy. That's for sure."

"I guess we both did the best we could Andrew. And I guess the best we could...stunk."

"Like someone with chronic physical pain, they come to accept their suffering as given and perceive it only when it increases beyond its normal intensity."

— Erich Fromm

Now, years after the injection …

"So, how often do you hurt?"

"I hurt all the time."

"But not a lot."

"A lot."

"But you don't hurt right now?"

"I hurt right now."

"You know you just don't look like a person in chronic pain."

"You know, I look exactly like a person in chronic pain."

I've wondered since the injection just what was expected of me. I remember the defense attorneys invested in proving that I wasn't dealing with all of this in a rational, appropriate manner. That I married at eighteen, and statistically teen marriages have a terrible success rate. That I refused medications, and I left my husband. And that for a four month period I drank alcohol daily.

But I also had a negligent injection, wound up in continual, horrible pain as a result of it, was mistreated and misdiagnosed by doctors that didn't want to be involved in a lawsuit, and was locked up in a psychiatric ward.

Did my choices contribute to my downfall, or my recovery?

Even now, years later, my anger still surfaces at unexpected times. I'm generally not aware of it, and at times I'm sure that the anger has exhausted itself. But at unexpected moments something will trigger it, and the anger will all come rushing at me.

I've been told that this whole experience matured me. It did that. I'm different now. I'm serious. I'm driven.

I live more fully than I did. And so the inevitable question is often asked, "Given all you've learned since the injection Kathleen, aren't you really better off now?"

And the answer varies. There are those days when things feel right, when I do not feel stressed beyond reason, when I feel fully alive, and I feel somewhat smug that I've made lemons into lemonade.

But sometimes I come across a photo of the pre-injection days, one that captures the old Kathleen. A photo in which I look happy and silly and relaxed.

And I remember when I didn't have a constant stabbing, cramping, viselike pain where I had the injection. Or a frequent dripping feeling down my left leg, a sensation I have yet to get used to, and that always leads me to quickly reach down with a feeling of embarrassment.

I remember a day when I didn't have to turn a certain way in the shower to prevent the water from spraying where I had the injection.

I remember when my day didn't start out with Tylenol and diaphragmatic breathing, and when I didn't have to be careful about seams or specific fabrics rubbing where I had the injection. When my left leg had as much feeling as my right, and I didn't have to be certain to step down from a step or curb or out of the car with my right leg first, or otherwise fall.

I remember when the temperature of my legs and buttocks felt the same on both sides, not on fire on the left.

I remember when I had a sickness barometer. Now on particularly bad days I can't tell whether I need to push myself to keep going, or whether I'm coming down with the flu and need hot soup and to fall into bed. I can't tell whether I am emotionally worn because of real life issues or because depression follows chronic pain.

I remember when I didn't have headaches most of the time, my jaw didn't click and throb, and physical therapy wasn't a given. When I didn't feel the guilt of hurting and failing my family.

But most of all I think about the years I lost with the girls and the innocence they lost so early. I think of how long it's taken for them to regain some sense of childhood, in which they could play and not be perfect. To believe that I would not wind up back in the hospital, and that they had nothing to do with my previous time there.

That's what I really want back, the time I lost with the girls. I want to take them down the slide on my lap again and see them laugh and beg me "one more time mommy, just one more time." I don't like to remember how I stopped picking up Amanda and lessened my carrying of Acasia because I couldn't take the chance that they'd touch me right where I had the injection, and set everything off. I don't like to think about the girls visiting me in the psychiatric ward, looking around, wide-eyed, silent, sad.

I can still hear the door closing when they left. Closing and locking.

I can't recover the years I lost with the girls.

But today the girls are beautiful and happy and healthy.

And me?

I still have chronic pain, but they were right at the pain clinic. I *can* control the bothersomeness. And Randy moved to California less than two months after we said good-bye in D.C. He proposed to me at the Bel Air Hotel with plane tickets "to Philadelphia to meet my parents" pulled out of one pocket, and a diamond and emerald bracelet, "I didn't want to pick a ring without you," out of the other.

Me??????? I stared at him in total disbelief. "In Washington I figured you didn't know what it's like to be with a person in chronic pain—the moodiness, the financial aspect, and ..."

"Kathleen, I want to spend the rest of my life with you and Amanda and Acasia," he interrupted smiling. "Not despite your pain but because of who you've become in dealing with it. You have the wisdom of someone who has successfully made it back from hell. You know what's important in life—and what isn't. We'll be great together," he said taking me in his arms.

And we are.

I see so many possibilities for life now. I have great plans. High hopes.

As for my latest anecdote, the one that keeps me going this week, it is from Stephen Nachmanovitch's wonderful book, *Free Play* —

"A story is told of a French railroad passenger who, upon learning that his neighbor on the next seat was Picasso, began to grouse and grumble about modern art, saying that it is not a faithful representation of reality. Picasso demanded to know what was a faithful representation of reality. The man produced a wallet-sized photo and said, 'There! That's a real picture—that's what my wife really looks like.' Picasso looked at it carefully from several angles, turning it up and down and sideways, and said, 'She's awfully small. And flat.' "

It works for me.

"May you live all the days of your life."

—*Jonathan Swift*

Acknowledgments

There were many people that made a difference to me during the years *The Day Room* takes place. Many of their names are included in this book, although the book could have been twice as long and still not given a glimpse into the comfort, support and constant love given to me by my mother, Peggy Crowley and my precious daughters, Acasia and Amanda.

In addition, I would like to thank —

All of my hospital buddies.

Ken Finger, a med student, for his insight, sensitivity and kindness.

Graeme Keeping for his editorial insight.

Larry and Jacqueline Schwartz for a thoughtful stream of information during my trial.

Gerilyn Karatsonyi for her belief in this book.

Gil Havas for his morning good cheer.

My ex-husband, Andrew Waddick. Things ended badly between us. But that doesn't change, nor will I ever forget, all that Andrew did for me, or how I once loved him.

The law firm of Bird, Marella, Boxer, Wolpert & Matz for a second Christmas bonus when the first was stolen.

Mark Drooks for his kindness, great taste in friends, and for lending his car to Randy. It was our first date, and Randy's first stickshift.

Sharai, just because.

My father, Ernie Crowley, for his critique and passion for life.

And most of all, my incredibly wonderful gift from heaven husband, Randy Stratt. He believed in me, Amanda, Acasia and *The Day Room* from the start. Women are now taught not to wait for Prince Charming, because fairy tales don't exist. But from the day I met Randy, I began living one.

Selected Bibliography

Below is a list of books (and one magazine) that I recommend. Many of these are available on audiocassette.

Alternative Medicine: The Definitive Guide. *Compiled by The Burton Goldberg Group. Puyallup, Washington: Future Medicine Publishing, 1994.*

Balch, James. F., M.D. and Balch, Phyllis A., C.N.C. Prescription for Nutritional Healing. *Garden City Park, New York: Avery Publshing Group, 1990.*

Borysenko, Joan. Minding the Body: Mending the Mind. *Reading, MA: Addison-Wesley Publishing Co., 1987.*

Chopra, Deepak. Quantum Healing. *New York: Bantam Books, 1989.*

Cousins, Norman. Anatomy of an Illness. *New York: Bantam Books, 1979.*

Fox, Arnold, M.D. and Fox, Barry. D.L.P.A.: To End Chronic Pain and Depression. *New York: Pocket Books, 1985.* (new printing scheduled for 1996)

Kabat Zinn, Jon. Full Catastrophe Living. *New York: Delacorte Press, 1990.*

Mind, Body Medicine: How to Use Your Mind for Better Health *Yonkers, NY: Consumer Reports Books, 1993.*

Mindell, Earl. Vitamin Bible. *New York: Warner Books, 1991.*

Moyers, Bill. Healing and the Mind. *New York: Doubleday, 1993.*

Murray, Michael T. Natural Alternatives to Over-The-Counter and Prescription Drugs. *New York: William Morrow, 1994.*

New Age Journal (a monthly magazine). *Mt. Morris, IL: New Age Publications (815-734-5808)*

Ornish, Dean. Dr. Dean Ornish's Program for Reversing Heart Disease. *New York: Random House, 1990.*

Ornish, Dean. Stress, Diet and Your Heart. *Orlando, FL: Holt, Rinehart, and Winston, 1982.*

Piper, Watty (pseud.). The Little Engine That Could. *Platt & Munk Co.(New York: Putnam Publishing Group), 1954.*

Reader's Digest Family Guide to the Natural Medicine. *Pleasantville, NY: Reader's Digest Association, 1993.*

Sacks, Oliver. A Leg to Stand On. *New York: Harper & Row, Publishers, 1984.*

Siegel, Bernie, M.D. How to Live Between Office Visits. *New York: Harper Collins, 1993.*

Siegel, Bernie, M.D. Love, Medicine & Miracles. *New York: Harper & Row, Publishers, 1986.*

Siegel, Bernie, M.D. Peace, Love & Healing. *New York: Harper & Row, Publishers, 1989.*

Weil, Andrew, M.D. Spontaneous Healing. *New York: Alfred A Knopf, 1995.*

Index